I Haven't Been *Entirely* Honest with You

I Haven't Been *Entirely* Honest with You

MIRANDA HART

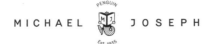

MICHAEL JOSEPH

PENGUIN MICHAEL JOSEPH

UK | USA | Canada | Ireland | Australia
India | New Zealand | South Africa

Penguin Michael Joseph, Penguin Random House UK,
One Embassy Gardens, 8 Viaduct Gardens, London SW11 7BW

penguin.co.uk
global.penguinrandomhouse.com

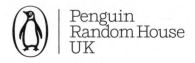

First published 2024
001

Set in 11.5/16pt FS Benjamin
Typeset by Jouve (UK), Milton Keynes
Printed and bound in Great Britain by Clays Ltd, Elcograf S.p.A.

The authorized representative in the EEA is Penguin Random House Ireland,
Morrison Chambers, 32 Nassau Street, Dublin D02 YH68

A CIP catalogue record for this book is available from the British Library

HARDBACK ISBN: 978–1–405–95833–2
TRADE PAPERBACK ISBN: 978–0–241–71887–2

www.greenpenguin.co.uk

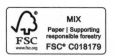

MIX
Paper | Supporting
responsible forestry
FSC
www.fsc.org
FSC® C018179

Penguin Random House is committed to a
sustainable future for our business, our readers
and our planet. This book is made from Forest
Stewardship Council® certified paper.

For You

Contents

A Prologue of False Starts

When I collapsed, I needed answers for what to do right there and then. It was a chronic situation, but it was still a crisis. I couldn't make myself a kale smoothie, or get to a yoga class, and I had no inclination to journal a gratitude list. I was ill and I was alone and I was debilitated. And I thought 'What do I do now?', 'How can I help myself right now?' And then there was a flicker of anger: 'There's a booming self-help industry out there, there's incredible awareness and discourse on holistic well-being from amazing experts, but I don't know what to do right now to help this critical moment of mine?'

I needed to know how to do the next ten minutes, and then hopefully the next. But I had nothing solid to draw on. No clear foundations to trust.

As the months went on, this made less and less sense. So, I thought, what are all the extraordinary scientists, neuro-scientists, psychologists, etc. today, mixed with ancient wisdom which many of them draw on, *actually saying*? What are the keys they all agree on? There must be universal truths to all the knowledge out there.

I decided to find out.

I needed to find out.

Because I needed to know how to do the next ten minutes . . .

Well, I did find out. I researched and studied and decided to write about it – which is why we are here My Dear Reader Chum (hello). But, I uncovered way more than I ever expected, so that I had absolutely no idea how and where to start this book.

Starting can be hard. Particularly with anything that feels significant.

It's rather bold to say this little book of mine feels significant because it may not feel that way to you reading the thing (hello again). For me, though, it's an epic embarkation. I'm putting to paper the depths of what I have discovered – and lived through – in recent years. I was not expecting my life to have turned out the way it has, or to unravel the way it did. But here I am, rather remarkably intact. And even more remarkably – certainly very surprisingly to me – with some answers that have led to living with a meaning, joy and freedom that I never thought possible.

My Dear Reader Chum, I had many attempts at starting this book. In the spirit of honesty, here are the different ways, and what I felt about them:

It's been quite the journey . . . *Oh no, very naff start. Start again . . .*

Roses are red, violets are blue, I'm going to have a cup of tea and hopefully do a poo . . .

Pull yourself together, Hart . . . Time to get serious . . .

Where's the life manual? Since my late teens I had never felt well. I had constant infections and injuries. If things improved or there was a moment of respite, I would be hit with another virus more debilitating than the last, slowly weakening my body year after year. Bronchitis, tonsillitis, pericarditis, costochondritis, gastroenteritis, labyrinthitis, too many 'itises' to mention; then a blood clot, slipped disc, ankle and knee ligament tears, adrenal fatigue, chronic migraines, parasites, cysts and blah blah blah blah BLAH. There weren't a few months, or even sometimes weeks, that passed without another 'itis' rearing its horrid head. In the end, every morning I woke up with a sense of dread of how on earth I was going to find the energy to get through the day. And I didn't know why it was all happening. Nor did the doctors who I was all too often passed between. It began to scare me. I felt like I didn't have the essential answers to all the brilliant science we now have on mind and body. I just felt overwhelmed. It seemed that I needed to read one book on mindfulness, another on sleep patterns, another on the mind–body connection, one on habits and goals and purpose, one on hormones, one just on dopamine, one on trauma, one on caffeine and one on alcohol – are caffeine and alcohol even acceptable? One person said yes, the other no, keep reading ... a book on power poses, one on ice baths, one on silent retreats, one on expressing your anger, another on soya beans. It was all too much. What were the basics to give me a starting point for change? Maybe I should write a manual ...

I don't think I can say I am embarking on writing a life manual for all humans, who do I think I am?! And, if you know

me at all, you know I'd only want to call it The Miranual . . .
Right, start again . . .

If you have ever heard the phrase 'coming home to yourself', have you, like me, felt some sense of peace, knowing it must be true, somehow, but having absolutely no blooming clue what it actually means? I delved around a bit for some answers. It was all a little confusing to start with – a lot of words like integrity and your false or shadow self versus your true self versus your ego versus your hairdo (I didn't know). I delved deeper and eventually settled on an exciting revelatory definition: 'Coming home to yourself: to operate from a place of peace and power, where you are free to be who you are (your authentic self) rather than buffeted by others' opinions of you or worldly measurements of success. Basically, utter self-acceptance.' Okay, yes, please, I want me some of that. Surely that's the key answer to being holistically well? Living as my true, wild self.

Oh dear, I believe that, but I end up sounding a bit grand and weirdly 'spiritual' . . . Start again . . .

Roses are red, violets are blue, sometimes I want to kiss a Beefeater, see what they'd do . . .

Let's pretend I didn't write that . . .
Apologies to you My Dear Reader Chum.
Okay, how about this . . .

As children we play, we explore, we stay in the moment, we shout 'look at me' without shame and show off a new skill, whether that's a twirl or a jump or a new toilet procedure, or all three at once (do try this at home). Then it slowly creeps in – the worry of what people think, the belief we must be 'cool' (whatever that means). We start to try, at all costs, to fit in. We lose our lovely playful part, possibly other parts too. And then we have a mid-life crisis and . . .

Hang on, I seem to have gone from twirling and farting to a mid-life crisis awfully quickly, though I appreciate twirling and farting could be symptoms of a mid-life crisis, the increase of the latter is certainly happening to me a lot, I veritably motor my way along . . . Moving on . . .

Roses are red, violets are . . .

Stop it . . .
I know, I'll start with a recent story . . .

To many, it would have been an ordinary moment in life. A dog walk. Donning some walking boots to negotiate a muddy path through a small wood. But I hadn't had much need for slippers in recent years, let alone walking boots, and I was beaming more widely than would be considered normal. Such a smile was also incompatible with the slippery mud under-foot; at the ripe old age of fifty, I'd suddenly become scared of falling over. (It happened almost overnight – now, I don't go to the bathroom without a phone in case I slip!)

Suddenly, the weight of this otherwise ordinary moment hit me. I saw a clump of bluebells. Again, nothing of earth-shattering importance to report. Except, you see, I'd been aching to see a bluebell wood for a very long time. Could I dare to hope that if I walked a little further, I might see the carpeted woodland floor I'd so longed to visit every spring for nearly a decade? I looked up beyond the clump that had stopped me on the path. There they all were; a blue hue cascading majestically down a steep bank towards a clear river. My breath was truly taken away. Indeed, I burst out crying!

The tears were for the sheer beauty of the bluebells, but also so much more. It had been precisely nine long years of waiting to be physically strong enough to see bluebells in spring. I cried, too, in acknowledgement of the last solid decade of ill health, and of how much my illness had taken from me throughout my life. I got 'all the feels', as I believe the young people say. She may be fifty but she's not out of the game, ladies and gentlemen! Still got her pulse very much on the cultural shizzle. (Anyone who has to profess this clearly does not, and, if I'm honest, until recently I thought Dua Lipa was a small family car . . .) So there, in my walking boots, on a muddy path with a carpet of bluebells before me . . .

Hang on, I seem to be starting my book at the end. I may not be the greatest literary mind, but even I know the best way to start a book might be from the beginning.

I think perhaps I am avoiding and therefore trapping myself to share truthfully from the start. Right, enough false starts, I have decided how to start. I will simply try and tell you my story.

We all have a story. I suppose that's what our lives are made up of: beautiful, unexpected stories of joy and despair, darkness and light, strength and vulnerability, in all their weird and wonderful guises. I know that I would not have been without the people – whether I've met them or not, whether they have been from completely different cultures and backgrounds or had completely different experiences – who have dared to share their stories, particularly their stories of pain and overcoming. I've felt connected, moved, heard, encouraged and informed by them. I don't know whether my story will do that for you, but I do believe I've learnt some useful nuggets along the way. Partly through negotiating some trickier times of my life and partly through what I call the 'ists': all the scientists, neuroscientists, therapists, psychologists, trauma specialists and sociologists we now have more access to and that I have read and watched and studied. And that's the point for me. I want to share the answers that were vital for my recovery – from long-term illness to living my life in a much more meaningful, free and joyful way. I suppose I'm writing the book *I* needed. And if you are still reading this . . . then I bid you a hearty hello – I think that's our third now, such fun! I hope that my story might help yours. Although as a dear friend of mine always reminds me when it comes to advice, 'Take what you want, leave the rest.'

Right, here we are. The actual start. Get yourself settled, My Dear Reader Chum. It's not a particularly jolly beginning, but there's nothing to fear. I'll be your cosy, warm comfort blanket (metaphorically, for I don't intend to knock on your door and smother my six-foot-one body all over you unannounced – sorry, it's gone weird). And spoiler alert, the book ends happily. So if you are digging in among any personal life difficulties at this moment, know that you can be okay. More than okay. You already are. You are fabulous. Fact. Whether you believe it yet or not.

Right, that's quite enough about you. Back to me . . .

PART ONE

Trapped

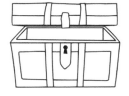

An Ending Was The Real Start

I knew it was pointless to call an ambulance.

I was alone and had just collapsed on to my sitting room floor, the worried licks of Peggy, my dog, trying her best to help me. I couldn't really move, such was the degree of exhaustion. I was genuinely concerned I might not get to the bathroom if I needed to go. I worked hard to lift my forearm off the floor so I could gently stroke Peggy in a bid to keep myself a little focused. I remember saying, 'It's very rare to die of exhaustion. I'm not okay, but it's okay,' trying to reassure Peggy as much as myself. I felt very weak. Like I didn't exist. Like I was fading away. Despite the severity of my fatigue (and it being the first time I had ever collapsed), I somehow understood that getting myself to hospital would be more of a stress than a solution. I knew enough about chronic ill health after three decades to know that my vitals would most likely register as normal, and that I would once again be sent home without clear answers.

Perhaps because I had nothing left to give, I wasn't scared. I was just sad. The emotion from years of wondering how I would make it through the day, of never really knowing why I was so exhausted, enveloped me like a heavy cloak. I just lay there. And waited. Either my body would start to come round or I would fade away. There was nothing I could do about it. I sank further into the rug and let out a long sigh. For despite the situation, there was relief. When you hit the end of the road, there is nothing left to do but let go. There are no longer choices of whether to go anywhere, whether to work, whether to push on. You're forced to just *be*, how you are, in the moment. And wait. In retrospect, moments like these – moments that people describe as the beginning of the end – can be celebratory. They are tales to be savoured and explored. What feels like the end is often a blessing in hefty disguise. In the moment, however, it's at best revealing and at worst completely horrific. I put mine towards the horrific end.

Immediately upon writing that I want to apologize and say I know how incredibly lucky I am and that I live with many privileges. I'm acutely aware of the desperate inequality and suffering held in this world. But I also believe that denying our stories out of guilt will only make them worse. Our grief and pain *are* allowed. Every story counts. With that, and the fact that my privilege compared with so many remains a deeply complicated, sad and difficult thing to hold in this world, I shall plough on.

The relief of hitting the end of the road began to morph into an overwhelming feeling of aloneness. In that moment, I didn't feel there was anyone I could call. How could I explain my fatigue? There was no clear diagnosis (that was to come years later). I felt (wrongly) that no matter who I rang, the telling of what had just happened would lead to too much worry, or not enough, or my being told that I was overreacting. Any judgement, any need to explain, any mis-understanding was too painful to risk.

4

After a few hours, thankfully, I could just summon the energy to crawl to the loo, followed dutifully by Peggy. I found myself in uncontrollable tears – partly in relief that I'd been able to move, but partly because I was faced, even more starkly, with how I felt. I told myself that all I could do was try to sleep and rest for a few days, and take it from there. I took it breath by breath as I slipped in and out of not consciousness, although it partly felt like that, but ghostly, inexplicable fatigue, a sluggish awareness, and significant pain as if my skin was on fire – yup, it was all truly delightful.

After four days I still felt like a ghost. Hollow. Nonetheless, I was so used to finding ways to keep calm and carry on – or at least just carry on – that I gathered my remaining strength to stay with my friends as planned. Particularly as it was Christmas and I didn't want to feel further alone. And because they were some of the trusted few to whom I could tearily announce on arrival, 'I feel horrendous and I don't know why. I'm a bit scared. Can I just be in a ball?' They smiled kindly and said, 'You're here with total acceptance and love, however you are.' A perfect script.

That Christmas, everything I felt internally bubbled away ferociously in stark contrast to the twinkly lights and jolly music of the season. I just tried to keep going, tried to find some lightness. Looking back, it's striking that I felt I had no choice but to keep going. So much of my life had been this way. No one had any answers for me. Doctors would tell me, after various tests would return as inconclusive, that it was probably stress or anxiety. Over and over again they would try to prescribe antidepressants, despite my not relating to

5

their diagnosis or having a clear understanding as to why the medication would help. I began to get angry that my body was letting my love for life down. I was full of dreams and desires, but my body felt under siege. The constant infections and viruses had weakened me considerably – just bunging antibiotics and anti-inflammatories at them (all the antis for the itises) was not sustainable as the years went on. I was constantly having to say no to things that I so wanted to do, or wasn't able to do them freely, fully or joyfully.

I was in a battle, and I wasn't winning.

I made a decision. This collapse, this end, had to be the beginning. The beginning of getting some answers, of getting my health back to where I had space and energy for excitement, for possibilities, for a future without pain. I lay in bed, the soft fur of my beloved dog next to my arm, the distant noise of my friends' sing-along I so longed to join echoing some cheer into my room, and I chose to believe that this could be my catalyst.

This end would be my real start.

The Sliding Cat

When I first experienced that collapsed moment at home, it was dusk. I was lying on my front, head facing towards the garden, and I could see the sky fading. I decided to heave my body on to my back so that I could watch that particularly

6

majestic English winter sky go fully dark through the skylights above me. It felt quite the feat: not just the physical effort, but the idea of facing my situation head-on rather than burrowing – literally and metaphorically – into my sitting room carpet.

I was given a great gift in doing so.

As I turned over, my neighbour's large tabby cat jumped on to the brickwork at the bottom of the skylight windows. It decided to make its way up to the roof, something I suspect it had done before, but not on a cold day with some remaining frozen pockets on the glass. This bulbous cat scrambled three-quarters of the way up the icy skylights with much comedic pedalling, but to no avail – the surface was too slippery. It was trying to maintain its dignity but simply could not get a purchase! The dear cat had to concede that it would not win this fine battle. It flopped on to the glass, like a Garfield toy squished flat against a car window and slid very slowly down. Our eyes met. Me, smiling, despite my situation (if I'd had the energy, I would have been really laughing), and the cat, looking in equal measure humiliated and furious. Making it, of course, even funnier. I wasn't laughing *at* the dear cat – I've done similar stunts in my personal and professional life – it just happens to be the kind of thing that makes me laugh, a lot. And laughter is a surefire way to true joy, I find.

This little moment, in which I could muster a smile despite everything, showed me that there can be treasures in darkness. My Dearest Reader Chum, I do really believe joy can exist even in our lowest moments. If we're bold enough to search for it, it will be there, whether it's a friendly smile, a falling leaf, a hot cup of tea or the most gracious surprise of a comedic animal.

My mind stirred. If I found this treasure on one of my hardest days, dare I consider that there could be more? That there could be an armour for and answers within darkness?

Darkness

I had been led to believe that dark moments were to be fought against, fixed, feared. Whether that darkness was illness, grief, a difficult work situation, an argument or just a mild hour of worry about something mundane, my reaction was the same. 'This is not on,' a voice within would shout in my sternest, posh, army-colonel-slash-boarding-school-matron voice – enjoy that image. I would be cross that I was feeling in some way weak or experiencing a less socially acceptable feeling. Aren't we always meant to be happy and positive and uncomplaining? That was my script, as it is for many of us. But as we continue this trip together, My Dear Reader Chum (or MDRC, if I may . . . for I already feel we are friends), I will show you what a lot of total garbage I now believe this is.

While I now know that joy is always there, I also know that darkness is part of life. Darkness is allowed. We're allowed to feel, and naturally will experience sadness and disappointment, fear and anger, embarrassment, and go from hysterical laughter to panic within the same day. And when we allow those feelings, the fear of them and of our difficult

experiences lessens. I could not have changed and trans-
formed if I had ignored the darkness (as you will discover, I
definitely tried!).

I realize that this is, of course, very easy to say, especially
in hindsight. We've still got to go through it.

The end, my rock-bottom, might have been the beginning,
but it was going to be a few more years of difficulty – of
darkness – to get to the other side.

The Cave

I will never forget a powerful image that came to mind a few
weeks after collapsing. I was in a rather bleary-eyed state,
and so I fear there's a chance this only makes sense to me, but
I'm diving in. Stick with me, in case you like the metaphor
that comes.

The image was of me on a path facing a very large boulder
that entirely blocked the way forward. For a while, I'd been
trying to push it out of the way or climb over it, but attempts
to do so only led to further exhaustion. I eventually had no
choice but to stand face to face with it. (This is when it gets a
little more surreal, and I probably only let my mind wander
because, well, when you're stuck in bed and the highlight of
your day is deciding whether to wash or get to the fridge, you
might as well . . .)

After looking at the boulder for a long time, thinking of it
only as my nemesis, a ruinous block on my path of life, I

started to approach it with a little more curiosity. I noticed that it had the shape of a door etched into it. I gently pushed the door, ready to step into whatever might be inside. It was dark. Musty. Dank. A cave. With slimy, muddy walls. I walked along the cold, rocky floor until another door at the far end of the cave became faintly visible. Somehow, I knew that door was one that I would eventually, at the right time, be able to step through. And I would be refreshed. The strength and knowledge needed for the journey out would stay with me, allowing me to live the rest of my life more fully. I know, MDRC (My Dear Reader Chum, lest you have already forgotten – RUDE), it's a lot. All I can say is that it felt somehow practical. And sensible.

What if, I thought to myself, it was time to stop fighting my body? Certainly, after years of trying to avoid and fix, I didn't have any fight left in me. What if the only way out was to see what I might learn by facing the mystery of all I was feeling head-on? To go through the dark, dank, murky cave until I got to the door on the other side.

Could there be glimmering treasures on the cave wall? Answers? A manual perhaps?!

What if the person who opened the door at the other end of the cave was me – healthy, energetic me? I was longing to get that person back, and not just the me with renewed physical health; I needed to reclaim all the parts of myself I had lost from the longevity of my illness, or the parts of myself I had never had the chance to discover – if I was to become fully healthy again.

Okay, hello darkness, you have my attention. Although darkness, 'old friend' – I'm not quite sure I can get there just yet. Simon & Garfunkel song break, MDRC? See you in a minute . . .

Hidden

I have been lucky enough to experience the very humbling loveliness of being told by thousands of people that the character I played in my sitcom, *Miranda*, freed them to accept who they are. I was writing a character who was trying to fit into the world, who didn't yet have the confidence to express who she truly was. I had no idea that it would resonate on the scale it did.

Lots of people would tell me of their socially bumbling 'Miranda moments'. I am delighted to report I have just had my own. Miranda's Miranda moment! I was in a doctor's surgery, and when my name was called, I didn't realize that my bag strap was caught round the arm of the chair I was sitting on. I walked towards the doctor with the chair screeching behind me, as if I had brought it as my pet. The doctor kindly but inadvertently patronisingly said, 'You don't need to bring your own chair!'

Comic moments aside, the resonance of *Miranda* also seemed to go deeper.

I remember being rather weepy when a young teenage girl wrote to me to say that she hadn't been going to school of late, for the bullying about being extremely lanky and tall.

Seeing 'Miranda' learning to cope with her height gave this young girl the confidence to put on her uniform one morning, fling her shoulders back and be determined not to mind any mean, snide comments that came her way. In fact, she said that with the new-found confidence in herself, the comments slowly stopped. I was very moved. There were others too – so many, actually – who told me that learning to accept themselves is what started to heal many other aspects of their lives.

Reflecting on this, in my moment of darkness, I considered again, particularly with the revelatory definition of 'coming home to yourself', that many of us dear humans likely feel trapped, knowingly or unknowingly, by the world and our experiences and what they can wrongly lead us to believe about ourselves. Our real, true, healthy, energetic selves hidden.

And then I focused on an assuredly less comedic way of considering this. I had read, in palliative care worker Bronnie Ware's book, *The Top Five Regrets of the Dying*, that the top regret was, 'Wishing I had the courage to live life true to myself, not the life others expected of me.' That broke my heart, MDRC. We *can* become hidden.

Hidden by parental and family expectation instead of following our own passions. Hidden by embarrassment, shame or shyness instead of voicing our opinions, or ending or forming relationships. Hidden by always trying to fit in and follow the crowd. Hidden by focusing on achievements and doings instead of discovering who we are and feeling good about and developing our personality. Hidden by a fear of not looking 'right' instead of boldly claiming our unique beauty. The list could be a long one: all the ways we mask who we truly are.

We are shaped by our family, by our relationships, by the places we live, the groups we belong to, the stories we tell ourselves or were led to believe. But these things can drive us to hide our glorious unique true selves.

If we think we are ugly, we hide our beauty.

If we think we are stupid, we hide our intelligence, our innovations, our imagination.

If we believe we shouldn't be weak or vulnerable, we hide from asking for the help we need.

If we believe we are defined by our job status, we keep striving and working and producing, and hide our playful, spontaneous, joyful selves, rarely resting.

If we have been led to believe our opinion doesn't count, or is foolish, we will become small to keep the peace.

If we believe our past failures identify our future, we hide our next ideas and our unique personality.

This certainly woke me up. And, if I was going to be honest with myself, (and you, MDRC), I had to face the surprising truth that, in some ways, I too wasn't wholly free.

And so, I set off with a purpose. I wanted to understand all the ways that life might have hidden the real me. I decided that I wanted to use this felled time of illness, this time in the metaphorical cave, to leave any habits and traits that didn't serve me in the past. I wanted to find the me that had been there before culture, the so-called right worldly ways, and life experiences changed me. Above all, I felt instinctively that these things could be contributing to my illness. That it was somehow all connected.

I was ready to step into the cave and learn.

Fame

Before I continue onward with my story, a quick aside, if I may. I know, we've only just begun, so please do very much bear with. This aside is about the f-word. And I do believe it's more of a curse than the usually described f-word. As I like to say, nothing like a good 'fuck' from time to time. Sorry!

But fame – it's quite the beast. The reason I mention it here is because I want to be clear that any exhaustive collapse I was experiencing was nothing to do with a lifestyle that can often be projected on to people possessing a degree of fame. I remember once being photographed at Wimbledon and a paparazzi asking me, slightly aggressively, to take my sunglasses off, which I didn't. He teased me: 'Ha ha, clearly a big night last night!' It was not said with a cheery tone, more a snide assumption that I was hiding bloodshot puffy eyes caused by a heavy consumption of alcohol. I thought, wow, even a middle-aged woman who advocates galloping can get tarnished with the brush that I was no doubt out partying and drinking until the early hours because I'm 'famous'. When 99 per cent of the time I am watching TV, bathing or snacking, often at the same time. In this instance, I didn't take my sunglasses off because I experienced symptoms at times that were caused by light sensitivity. Plus, I'd done my eye make-up very badly, and I thought there was a risk that I might look like I was doing a bad Alice Cooper impersonation.

There were certainly aspects of my job that contributed to exhaustion (fame is a trap in itself). But illness would have happened anyway.

Whilst we are here, may I say, for the record, that I would certainly not recommend fame. It's a strange creature. Even if it's something that you aspire to – which I declare as foolhardy – it is not in your control as to whether it happens. It is put upon you. It happens because you have a moment of popularity (or notoriety). And that popularity isn't your fault! You're just doing something you do, doing a job, and you can't help it that people decide to like you and it leads to fame. And then all it does is take. Fame is not a friend, it's a taker. The system that desired to make you famous wants equally to tear you down, seemingly with glee. Like a kindly grand-parent telling you how lovely you are and giving you a gift, and the next day screeching that you are a piece of shit (sorry to do a shit at you, as it were) and didn't deserve the present. It's very confusing.

I didn't bristle against any fame or critique. I enjoyed the ride, taking it all with a pinch of salt. In some ways, I believe it's a good thing that I ended up with some fame. For instance, I once very nearly whipped my clothes off and jumped into the Trafalgar Square fountain on a hot day. But I resisted, as no one wants to see that kind of naked honesty on their social media over breakfast. Moving on . . .

It's important for people to remember that fame is not

a joy-giver. It's not the gift of a sliding cat. I think there's only *one* good thing about fame. And that one thing is better customer service. (But even that comes with a sting because it's irritating that there isn't good customer service *for all*.)

Kids, let me say this: if you see a happy famous person, the reason they're happy in that moment is not because they are famous. Unless they've just received super customer service.

So, no, there was no rock-and-roll lifestyle that led to exhaustion for this comedy actress. I refer the honourable reader to the aforementioned 'night out' consisting of wallowing in a bath with snacks.

The Elephant

Talking of wallowing, if I had to name my favourite animal, it would be the emotionally astute, glorious elephant. One of my happiest memories is of washing one with a broom in a muddy river as it wallowed and rolled when I visited a sanctuary in Thailand. But my tale of elephants here gets a little less cheery. To say the least. Buckle in.

Reflecting on the concept of our true selves being hidden, I believe I now know why I reacted so violently – so viscerally – to a video at the sanctuary about how the elephants they rescue are captured. When captured, wild elephants are put in tight, wooden cages. They can barely move, and every time they roar, scream or try to break down their shackles to

free themselves back to the wild, magnificent, feeling creatures that they are, they are prodded by a human who has
fashioned a sharp, wound-inflicting blade at the end of a long
stick. Eventually, after days of this, an elephant knows there's
no hope. It realizes that if it is quiet and still, it won't get hurt.
It has been beaten into submission. This elephant must forget
who its young, wild self was.

As the humans remove the wooden cage, they tie up the
elephant's feet with chains. If it runs, it will fall. It can only
lumber listlessly, at a pace slow enough so that the chains
don't cause a damaging crash to the ground. Eventually it
becomes a slave to its human boss. A wild animal working in
a tourist industry. People will pay to receive bananas and
bags of peanuts from her. She's terrified. By the noise. By the
lights. She's a wild animal in a world that isn't hers. But she
can't show her fear. She has had to stop being truly alive in
order to survive.

It's a distressing and intense picture. We're horrified, not
just because of the terrible, appalling animal cruelty but
because, I believe, there might be some resonance for our
own lives, too. Many people have experienced, to extremely
varying degrees, moments of being abused, of being told to
shut up, of being forced to make decisions against their will,
of having their rights ignored. We might all, to some degree,
however seemingly innocent and perhaps unknowingly, have
been pushed and prodded by people and systems that aren't
in our best interest.

And that's what I meant earlier, when I mentioned 'so-
called right worldly ways'. If you want to come on this

adventure with me, MDRC (and thanks for still being here – I can promise it gets jollier as we go on), then you should know that if I say 'the world' had taught me to feel or be or do a certain way, then I mean contemporary culture, the rules, practices and trends we have been led to believe are true.

Worldly 'rules' that shout things like be nice and polite at all costs, because being nice and polite is what gets you places; get good grades even if you aren't academic; don't express any embarrassing emotions; be outgoing and funny and fascinating as that's the only way to 'succeed' socially; know exactly what you want to do, have a career path mapped out and put huge pressure on yourself to have a job that makes you look and sound successful; be petite and sweet and feminine if you're a woman, and for goodness' sake don't be too loud, opinionated or angry, yet take up your space and grab success; try not to wrinkle or age and shift your face to stay young; fit in to make sure you have a 'cool' group of friends; get on the property ladder or live in a camper van or tiny house, nothing in between because you don't want to be boring; but don't be weird; don't just be a stay-at-home parent, also run a business or a charity, but look after the children perfectly so that they don't suffer any emotional issues; take lots of rest and spend money you don't have to go on amazing, photograph-perfect holidays, but also make sure you are really busy and constantly in very important meetings; keep proving you're a good person by meeting everyone else's needs because it's still selfish to look after yourself even though self-care is now common parlance. And on and on and on it goes. (And we haven't even mentioned the severity of trauma from racism, asylum-seeking, domestic violence, sexual abuse, dictatorships and all the stuff in the world that's so hard but necessary to look at.)

18

Rather a bleak picture – I told you it wasn't a pretty start. But I felt that by daring to listen to what I was feeling, by considering this idea of our real selves being hidden, I was already gaining some understanding. A hypothesis was forming. One I believed (and at the risk of sounding grand) might be an answer for others, too. Perhaps it could ease anxiety, or agitations and restlessness and discontent, sleeplessness, low-grade tiredness and tension, and hopefully beyond.

You see, what I'd already discovered by dipping into the 'ists' is that – get this – we are neurobiologically wired to belong. (Oh, and for those who weren't concentrating earlier or who don't read a prologue (again, RUDE), the 'ists' are all the scientists, neuroscientists, therapists, psychologists, trauma specialists and sociologists, etc. that I have learnt from via courses, their books and the kindness of their (often free) resources on YouTube, websites and social media. Thank you, 'ists'.) It's amazing, MDRC. We know – scientifically! – that we are wired for connection: to love and be loved. Love and belonging are essential for surviving, let alone thriving.

How exciting. Here was a clear link showing how hiding ourselves – trying to fit in by losing who we are – is *disastrous* for our holistic health and happiness. Life becomes a fascinating but troubling loop: we hide to fit in because we are wired to belong, BUT if we aren't belonging honestly as who we really are, we aren't belonging at all.

The 'ists' were saying that we therefore seek love and security by doing all we can to prevent anyone hurting us or shaming us. Maybe we're stuck in perfectionism or comparison or busyness or workaholism or people-pleasing. It's no wonder so many people are tired and anxious. It's no wonder the top regret of the dying is what it is. Many people end up protecting themselves by putting on masks that become exhausting to maintain as any masks we wear are, simply and truly, not who we naturally are.

I now feel much less idiotic for wanting to shake people at polite English social events and say, 'But what are you *really* thinking?' or 'What excites you?' or 'What saddens you?' or 'Let's TALK.' For wanting to whip my clothes off and run around between the seemingly uptight ties and frocks, throw creamy scones in people's faces and scream! Obviously I am not condoning this! I know that introductory small talk is welcoming, and kind, and a way for us to initially feel safe with each other. But I am someone who wants to tear down the curtain and see the real play as soon as possible. Take off the masks. See all the humanness. The brilliant and ridiculous. Terrified and tremendous. Loveable and laughable.

I feel sure all each of us wants is for others to see the real, wonderful us. And vice versa.

I want to see everyone's inner elephants!

Waiting And Longing

It's strange how hard waiting is. I have found that even waiting for a bus can be a deeply frustrating thing. (Me, impatient? What do you mean?!) I want to keep on schedule, for things to run as planned, and when the bus is late, I must wait. Get still for a moment. Feel the irritation. Possibly have to feel uncomfortable. Oh, how we hate feeling uncomfortable.

Waiting involves physical and emotional discomfort of varying degrees whatever the cause – a late bus or the drawn-out loss of a loved one, a three-day migraine or ten years of illness. Waiting is hard. It's not a gentle time-out. It's not a state of pleasure.

A few months after I collapsed, I remained in a period of waiting. Waiting for the energy to be more out of my bed than in it, waiting for medical answers, amongst others. I had to face another thing we humans don't appreciate: lack of control. In my waiting, I was no longer in control. I had no control of when or if I would recover, of when the grief might ease. None of us is in control of much. Of what time we will get to our destination, of which loved ones stay with us, of that job idea, of when we might get pregnant, or of what our children do. Of anything. But we try to maintain control to ease discomfort.

The hardest blessing in hefty disguise of being forced to let go of control, sit in the darkness and wait, was the discomfort caused by becoming aware of the depths of longing I had not felt before. I suspected that many of the things I wanted, or was acknowledging I didn't want to be without (perhaps on some level for the first time), were parts of that wild self that had been hidden. The stillness of illness (ooh, a pleasing little rhyme in a tricky time) led me to acknowledge head-on my then-greatest longing.

I didn't want to be alone anymore.

I confessed to myself that I wanted to find love and share my life with another. I admit, MDRC, it was harder than I imagined it would be to acknowledge this. Despite it being exciting and important to dream, sometimes, when it's admitting an innermost longing, it's scary to be faced with the current lack. It's why so many people give up on their dreams: it's hard to face what we don't have when we dare to long. And in this case, I now knew why the longing not to be alone can feel acute – we are literally wired to love and be loved. To belong.

But I believed listening to the longings in my waiting would be worth it. I felt sure it would be part of coming home to who I truly am. Meeting that wild self before the world got at her. That would assuredly make going through the darkness worth it.

True Identity

Right, I thought. What exactly is this wild self? It's easy to spout in a pseudo-spiritual way but I didn't want to leave any stone unturned on this journey through the cave. It led to me considering the whole concept of identity.

I was humbled by an illness that made me house- and bed-bound on and off for a long time. That meant I could no longer create who I was by any of the usual measurements. Over the years, I lost not only my health but my job, my independence, my friendships, my hobbies, my physical strength, my mental energy and my concentration. Even my house. I will tell all as we go along, but suffice to say I was humbly stripped bare.

I looked up a definition of identity: 'The qualities, beliefs, personality traits, appearance and/or expressions that characterize a person or group. Identities are strongly associated with roles or the group memberships that define the individual.' To that end, who we are and what we become are influenced as we identify by age, gender, race, religion, skills, education, political affiliation, careers.

Yes, but . . . what goes below that? Oh yes, MDRC, this waiting was giving me much pause for thought. It was an intriguing moment. To be stuck in bed, with none of the Western world's trappings of 'success' or identity. Just a person. Just me. Perhaps I was truly experiencing that too for the first time. I didn't know. But I did feel that if our identity is wholly made up of our looks, jobs and other external identifications, then we must be missing a beat. Who are we at our core? What unites us all?

And then it clicked. I was slowly catching on! If every single human being has the intrinsic need to belong, then isn't our core identity that we are simply loved and loveable for who we are? It would be easy to think the term 'wild self', that I have started to use from the arresting image of that dear elephant, means being another kind of person to who we actually are. I wouldn't want that term to lead you to believe you need to release an inner warrior, or tiger – to literally 'be wild'. No need to rip your clothes into shreds, and rage furiously, putting two fingers up to every aspect of society. (Although some of us will naturally be activists, advocates and change makers.) By wild self I mean, simply, who you are. You. Your loved and loveable authentic self. The majestic masterpiece that is you, whether you believe that (yet) or not. (I so hope my story does lead to that outcome – as I say, things do get jollier . . .) The one and only true you that could have become hidden unknowingly by the masks we can wear to fit in.

Oh gosh, now I was having an existential moment – do I know who I am, *really*, just me, just me here in this bed with nothing to be able to prove myself, no anecdote to regale with (apart from what snacks are best in and around a bath), no abilities as such in this moment? Perhaps all those worldly stabs can get to us so early on in our lives that we never get to know the wild creation we truly are. We don't realize we are never operating as our authentic selves.

And this made sense to me. Isn't every one of us, to some degree, looking for ways to heal insecurity, anxiety, fear, restlessness, confusion, jealousy and so on, by knowing we're loved and accepted?

If you truly believed you were inherently loved, accepted, approved, allowed – would there be any need to hide? Would there be any fear of being judged by others, thinking you are too much or not enough, not letting yourself follow a dream or an idea, any need to believe what bullies said about you, any fear of failure, or shame of going through difficulty and darkness? Surely all those trappings could slowly fade away? I knew that with an incapacitating illness, all I needed, more than ever, was to feel loved and accepted.

My purpose for this time gathered momentum. I was in an identity-less vacuum and I was going to fill it with a renewed sense of belonging and acceptability. I remembered a quote by holocaust survivor and psychologist Edith Eger in her extraordinary memoir *The Choice*: 'When we come to believe that there is no way to be loved and to be genuine, we are at risk of denying our true nature.' Wow, that really hit home. We hide ourselves out of fear that our real selves can't be loved.

Gosh, I am so done with the masks!

I'm just going to lighten the mood for a moment. I have been typing this in my dressing gown in the morning and I just went to let my dog out into the garden, still wearing only said dressing gown. The cord was trailing near the floor, and she grabbed it to play with it, thereby loosening my dressing gown. As we walked back into the house, the cord still in her mouth, she expertly peeled my dressing gown apart to reveal my naked body – it looked like a fully trained and rehearsed burlesque act! What would have just been amusing turned into a sitcom moment as, revealed in all my glory, I came face to face with the bin men at my kitchen window. I screamed and ducked as quickly as I could but let's just say it will be hard to look the bin men in the eye again . . .

Let's move quickly back to my philosophizing.

Suffice to say, I was excited, despite everything, because I came to believe that living from a rock-solid belief in our true identity changes everything. Instead of viewing statements like 'love yourself' and 'be your true self' as trite or naff or just a nice notion or a way to sell a cool t-shirt, if we could under-stand them scientifically and spiritually, they might be the foundation for holistic health and a joyful life. (Holistic was the key word for me, for I really wanted to know that I could have joy and meaning, even if I never recovered from what was ravaging my dear body.) The 'ists' I had read so far were saying as much. And those wonderful young people who told me they had freed themselves and got healthier from various conditions via my sitcom seemed like my inadvertent evidence.

We all know that long-term stress is the true killer. It's how disease manifests and grows within. I hypothesized further that a genuine sense of belonging and wholehearted love of who we are, truly accepting ourselves, could reduce many life stressors. Blimey, it was worth peeking into the cave entrance.

What Do You Need To Leave Behind?

I've always enjoyed a gentle wander through a graveyard. You might think that rather sinister or morbid, MDRC. But for me it's the opposite. I find graveyards beautiful, reflective and inspiring. Beautiful because namely I think about English church village graveyards set among flint and red brick, an old yew tree that holds the secrets of all that's gone before, robin song and the mossy, grey headstones. Reflective, as looking at the end of life, I'm always inspired to live mine to its fullest and freest before I move on. I become wistful about all I may have missed and regretted, but any sense of wasted time becomes inspiring.

For the things that make me deeply grieve if I look around a graveyard are not death and endings, for those are inevitable, but any unique dreams and regrets that might be buried in those plots. I hope each person was free to be who they were, follow the desires of their hearts, so they could give the world what it needed from them. I hope they loved how they were meant to love, and made the changes they were meant to make on whatever scale.

This led me to think about our individual identities. Yes, we all share the inherent design to be loved and to love, but the way we show love and the skills and personalities that make up the rest of our identity are all different. I remembered the time I looked at a particular gravestone, just as a blackbird rather romantically came to sit atop it and sing, and wondered what this person who had walked this earth, a century or so before was like. What they did, how they spoke, what brought them joy. Each of us, every person, is utterly unique.

Looking at a gravestone also jolts me into what's important – as I can't help but consider why I love and miss people. You're rarely going to hear a eulogy that includes, 'The thing I will miss most about them is their yogic core strength,' or, 'The main thing I loved them for was all their business awards,' or, 'The greatest gift they gave me was putting in that beautiful kitchen island and those new scatter cushions.' No, you will hear memories of that person making someone laugh, being generous, helpful, peaceful, playful, gentle. Memories of times of connection, compassion, joy, kindness, creativity.

How much we earned, what sort of people we met, what kind of accolades we received – they are all random, amusing, interesting additions, but not the reason we are loved.

Since *Miranda*, people often ask me for advice about how

they can feel happier in themselves. This has become my answer: Mull on the truth that there's only one of you in the whole history of humankind ever. No one who has come before you is the same. No one who has come after you is the same. You are the only you who has ever appeared in history, therefore you simply ARE valuable, needed, approved, accepted. You ARE loved. Plus, you have a set of DNA, skills, imaginations, visions and attributes that create a unique personality that the world needs at this time. That's your wild self! Just you.

And that's what my story is about. How I understood and left behind, or rather wholly smashed, old 'worldly' patterns that didn't serve me. But it is also a story of putting things on. Of picking up things lost from my past. Any habits or behaviours that felt like a trap that might be hiding a part of me, I would drop; all that sparked joy and peace and freedom and aliveness, I would pick up. Perhaps you also feel it's time to turn from and smash old patterns, to free yourself to leave behind a legacy that is your one beautiful life. As best as any of us can.

There's a lot to leave behind so that you can leave behind what you want to leave behind. (Pleased with that!)

Humble Superpower

I should add, being our wild self doesn't mean the need to become some kind of superhero or superstar.

In the classic movie set-up, someone turns their average

28

grey suit into a hero's cape with extraordinary powers no one else possesses. But the true superpower is being happy in the 'grey suit' – just who you are, because there's only one of who you are. You're allowed to be seen in all your ridiculous, broken glory. That's the point. You don't need a cape. You don't need to pretend to be strong. You don't need to offer what you think are your acceptable aspects and hide what you think is less desirable. Your own DNA is your superpower. Turning from the need to be superhuman into the everyday, perfectly imperfect you – that's your superpower.

Being wild means taking off the masks and living with a radical sense of authentic self, but you can still be an accountant!

Finally, Baggage Reclaim

I was nineteen and in the baggage reclaim of Heathrow airport on return from months travelling around Australia and New Zealand. One of the greatest and happiest experiences of my life. The reason why my memory of that otherwise tedious time in a municipally lit grey room – everyone fighting for their suitcases after a long flight among their weighty emotional baggage (pleased with that too) – came to mind didn't initially present itself, but as I sat with it, it developed and became clear.

I remembered, having collected my well-travelled rucksack, not going straight through to arrivals but sitting on a bench of grey, metal-backed seats. They were next to the automatic doors to arrivals, where my family were waiting on the other side to greet me and drive me home. I had started to walk towards the doors but just as they opened, I found myself diving, as if to safety, towards the seats. I hid. There was something in me that did not want to return. As the memory grew stronger, I remembered how trapped I had felt – like my true nature, which had been freed and allowed and expressed and in flow while travelling, was coming back to a place it shouldn't be, or couldn't function. I was rooted to the chair, thinking like a fugitive of how to escape. At the time I didn't know why this was happening. I felt guilty that I had a loving family and a home to go back to but was pinned in baggage reclaim with not an ounce of desire in me to return. It was as if my wild self was telling me that the plans that lay ahead, that the routines and habits of the life waiting for me, were indeed a trap, and simply not who I was designed to be. I was not interested in doing politics at university in Bristol, which was my next step and one of the first micro-stabs I can recall against my wild self. (I heard once that it isn't necessarily the big traumas that affect us over a lifetime but the constant microaggressions.)

I have very little memory of my time at university, but I do remember that in the first term, I took myself to London to do a day's interview for a stage manager course at Central School of Speech and Drama. I don't mind sharing, I came top of the class and got offered a place. It was my neat presentation in a new hardback folder on the Bristol Hippodrome, where I worked front of house, that sealed the deal – nothing like a bit of laminating to help impress. (I do love stationery!) Theatre had been my passion since I could remember. I would have absolutely loved to move from doing politics to a stage management course. Yet I sat on the train back to Bristol, keeping the whole thing secret, not wanting to rock the boat. (It seems a little mad to me now.) I didn't want to upset my parents or my teachers, and there was even shyness about admitting I wanted to go into the arts. I kept my dreams and passions hidden for a long time. I am intrigued as to whether these kinds of small ways we go against our nature lead to emotional and physical health problems and niggles. Perhaps it was no coincidence that before I finished my third year, I was heading back to my parents' house after many infections and viruses had first significantly weakened me.

I don't know how long I remained sitting in baggage reclaim. It felt like hours. I do remember eventually walking through the airport sliding doors with a heavy heart. That nineteen-year-old knew on some level that in Australia she had been free because she'd been unburdened of all that can unknowingly trap us.

If only we're honest. If only we listen. If only we know what to do when we listen. If only we have the opportunities to follow what we have heard.

I felt sure it was not too late. I could start again.

I was off to reclaim HER.

Starting Again

Shaking legs, unsteady
Like elastic stilts.
All new, each step funny and fragile,
But not new.
Not a tottering calf at birth
Nor a wobbly toddler
Or duckling slipping on ice.
New, but oh, oh so familiar.

Decades of walking, sprinting,
Rushing, rambling,
Sliding, jumping, skipping,
Dancing.
Runs now coming up half a century,
And she's out.

Imprisoned, locked down,
Shut in and shut up,
Lost, forgotten.
The strong and sturdy sticks
Fading backwards,
Inexperienced in weakness.

Unlearning the basics of before;
Time to walk once more.
So familiar, so foreign,
So frail, so fresh.
Ready to dart and dash,
Knowing nothing can be rash.

As the pins uncurl,
As the joints unfurl,
The steps are just that:
Single steps,
Minute and mammoth.

Where they will take her,
She does not know.
And with that thought,
On with the show.

– Me

PART TWO

Treasures

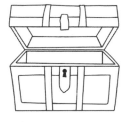

Treasure One

Share

TREASURES PICKED UP: Belonging, sharing, listening, connecting, gathering

PATTERNS SMASHED: Isolation, being a burden, invulnerability, not asking for help

WATCHWORD: Connection

SOUNDTRACK: 'The Shoop Shoop Song (It's in His Kiss)' by Cher

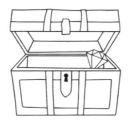

Share

A Silly Mood

I just made myself chuckle, imagining that those listening to the audiobook of my ramblings might think that the first treasure I discovered was the singer Cher. They might think, *Wow, strange, she went through a torrid time and a key answer was pop sensation, nay goddess, Cher. Are we going to be instructed to ritualistically dance to 'The Shoop Shoop Song'?*

Just to be clear to all of you listening half-heartedly to me while hoovering or driving (I jest, I love me an audiobook, and a hearty hello to you listeners), I mean 'share' as in S, H, A, R, E. Worth spelling out to us all, such is the importance of sharing. Not sharing everything, of course. I will not share food. Absolutely not. If anyone attempts to reach over and take a chip off my plate, they will be batted firmly away. Nor will I entertain the notion of 'can I just try yours?', and before I answer a fork is descending upon my plate. Absolutely not, thank you please. I chose what I'm having, you chose what you're having, and deal with it we must. Right, I've got that off my chest.

And this has served as a perfect example of using humour as a diversion from the vulnerability needed to share with another . . . I shall bravely go forth. Though not before another

41

quick diversion to say that I like the idea of Cher-ing as a verb to describe a group of Cher fans having a fabulous time.

Stop now, Miranda, and crack on with Treasure One, please, I hear you say . . .

And I will. Because sharing and connection, and all I learnt about them in this first glistening treasure, is more crucial than I ever knew. Although, and I promise this is the last diversion . . . it seems wrong not to have a quick, stress-busting dance break. Feel free to join. Obviously, it would be churlish not to choose Cher. I'm off to Shoop Shoop . . .

A Problem Halved

That was a thrilling bop! It transported me back to my school life. Always a happy place for me to go to. I know I'm unusual in that my school days really were among some of the best days of my life. For years I used to wonder why I missed school quite so much. In particular, being part of a sports team. It was where and when I was at my happiest: sharing a common goal with my teammates, wanting to better ourselves with each other's help. Nothing beats that. Perhaps I missed my true calling, and I was meant to have been a professional lacrosse player or a PE teacher – I can just imagine myself galloping Penelope Pitstop style up and down a pitch using my whistle with gay abandon! Quite the image . . .

What I've come to understand is that I was missing the true and deep connectedness that comes when you are part of a team. And that as an adult, I had unknowingly drifted further and further away from that particular kind of natural community and connection. I went from being a solid teammate to experiencing the detriment of isolation. I became less and less practised in sharing difficulties (and perhaps this was never practised enough – a vital thing we aren't necessarily taught), or, rather, completely conditioned out of) so that when my big crisis came along, it felt easier to keep the problem to myself.

If I heard the expression 'a problem shared is a problem halved' I would feel instantly irritated. It made no sense to me. I was more of the belief that a problem shared is a problem doubled: a problem dealt with alone will surely go away without the need to burden another.

But when I began to sit with what I'd learnt about our identity, I understood why we're not meant to be alone. When we know that the essential part of our humanness is the need to be loved and to belong, we also know that we're not helping ourselves when we don't deeply connect or share. It doesn't make it easy, but I found it made it a little easier to know it's what I have to do to be healthy.

If we're designed to be loved and connected, then it's an assault on who we are to not be heard. And we can't be fully heard if we don't share our problems. It's an assault on ourselves and our loved ones not to be honest.

My ache for the interconnectedness, camaraderie and ready-made social life of my school days really spoke to that.

And indeed, there have been many studies on the effects of loneliness, and stark evidence that it increases the risk of illness. In fact, a contributing factor to trauma after a distressing incident is often put down to the lack of a kind or loving witness to help in that moment. Big stuff.

Being seen and accepted without judgement is a fundamental human need.

Yet so often we bottle up and don't give people the opportunity to help us.

Why is it so blooming hard?! Why did I rile so much against 'a problem shared is a problem halved'? It seems strange to me now that I did, but the forces at play that made it easier to disconnect were strong.

Right, it was time to look at those forces, the patterns I needed to smash, if I was to become connected and feel the health and goodness of being a teammate again.

We Are Not A Burden

I'm using the 'royal we' here, MDRC, because I feel pretty sure that I'm not alone in holding the fear of being a burden. I know only too well how easy it is to go it alone, for I spent many years shouldering my burdens myself.

It turned out I was more burdensome in my fear of burdening another! I was only becoming more tired, more unwell, more anxious by not sharing. Our friends and family will worry more, not less, when we don't let them in. Sadly, the plain fact is it's harder to be loved if we don't ask for help.

And there's our answer. Because we are wired to be loved, and connectedness is necessary to survive, let alone thrive, it can be a terrifying concept to us to share – because, what if we are rejected? So strong is the need for love and connection that the fear of not having it makes it easier to hide.

Of course people don't share lest they be misunderstood or judged, for that's our greatest fear. (It's why I didn't call anyone the day I was lying on my sitting room floor in an exhaustive collapse. I just wanted to be held and heard, but that was not part of my culture. Yet.)

So, the masks come on. Off we go pretending that we're absolutely fine, so as not to burden each other. 'How are you?' 'Oh, really well, thanks.' 'Are you sure . . . you're limping and your leg doesn't seem quite right?' 'I think I just broke it falling down those steps, but I'll fashion a crutch from a twig and crack on – someone's coming for dinner and I can't let them down. Onwards and upwards!'

I shouldn't jest, for it is one of the things I find so very sad in this world. By masking, we move further away from ourselves and each other and that connection our health needs, despite it being for the seemingly good reason of avoiding rejection. There's an extraordinary quote by author and theologian Frederick Buechner, who says we become an 'edited version which we put forth in hope that the world will find it more acceptable than the real thing'. A heartbreaking notion, I find.

If, like me, you want some statistics to back up the idea of the need to belong as part of our identity, then there are many out there, but I would like to give you my version of the science called: 'The Mess of a Break-Up'. Simply, why else do we crumble so readily when we break up with a friend or a partner? We truly can crushingly crumble, can't we? I put it to you, MDRC, that if relationships weren't so important, then we wouldn't naturally crumble. (I am enjoying the word crumble.) Last time I crumbled, I did it literally and metaphorically as I wept my way through a series of actual crumbles. FOR DAYS. The excuse I gave was that I was tasting the variety of crumble puddings and toppings available, to find the perfect combination. I convinced myself that I'd been appointed this vital job for the nation by the Queen. Royal Crumble Taster. Otherwise, I was just a woman in her forties listening to romantic ballads, snotting uncontrollably into a crumble.

The sometime ridiculousness of break-ups proves clearly to me the vital, human need for connection. Although I briefly questioned why on earth I had even contemplated that deepest longing, to open the Hart heart up to love. It felt grossly vulnerable to dare to consider romantic love after years of being single. To consider someone really getting to know me, warts and all. (I don't have warts.)

Trouble is, the longer we leave it to connect in the way we need to, the harder it can be. Holding it together ourselves and not burdening anyone seems like a show of strength, but it's really frightening to be and to feel too alone. I learnt something fascinating and vital from the wonderful 'ists' – our nervous system needs a sense of dignity to feel safe and therefore function efficiently. What a heavy revelation, MDRC, that we can be in biological, physical stress when we're not regularly dignified by connection to a person who holds every part of us with respect and kindness. Disconnection is an unnerving experience even on a cellular level.

When I learnt that a felt sense of dignity was my right and what I needed for a fully functioning brain and body, I began to truly hope I could get back to deep connection. This time without being on a lacrosse field – I don't think I'd feel dignified if the menopausal mounds (code for mahoosive middle-aged bosoms) were forced to bounce ferociously up and down a sports pitch. Though I could use them defensively – I'd whack people in the eye with them . . . Moving on . . .

Of course, there are some people for whom vulnerability and sharing are naturally part of their lives, and they know them to be the bedrock of wholehearted, healthy living – they simply won't understand those of us who are trying not to be a burden. They may say to us, 'Yes, it can be icky and tricky to make that step to ask for help, share a secret, admit an issue, address a relationship problem, start dating again, but what's the alternative?' To which I would happily say, 'Oh, that's easy, good old-fashioned emotional repression, keep calm and carry on, if you want a job done do it yourself, being needy is weak and asking for help is embarrassing and pathetic, that is what the world has told us so we are scared and scarred to share, thank you please to you please!'

As I read Brené Brown's research on the matter, I knew I had to change these ways: 'Connection is the energy that exists between people when they feel seen, heard and valued; when they can give and receive without judgement; and when they derive sustenance and strength from the relationship.' She also wrote, 'Chronic disconnection leads to social

47

isolation, loneliness and feelings of powerlessness. Disconnection can cause people to lose touch with their own feelings and inner experiences.'

TATT

I've seen countless doctors over my time. There have been some positive experiences of kindness and empathy, but in the main, they saw I wasn't dying, couldn't understand my cluster of symptoms, and didn't really help beyond saying, 'I'm sure a week or two of rest and you'll be fine.' When you try resting for weeks every few months and nothing changes, that gets a little wearisome. However, there was one experience of doctoring that was more scarring.

I was in a doctor's office, sharing with him that I felt desperate for answers for the degree of fatigue and muscular pain I had to live with. It was at a time when work was beginning to go quite well. I'd been able to give up temping in offices and could now call myself a professional actor, getting small parts in sitcoms. I was concerned that my body wasn't going to cope with these opportunities I'd worked hard for and was excited to have. I of course didn't waste the doctor's time with my history of trying to get into comedy, but I was quite plainly and calmly saying that my life was being hugely hindered. I was still getting virus after virus with little gap in between, I didn't know anyone else at my age who was struggling in a similar way, and I wanted to investigate, so as not to risk the chance of giving up on work that was so meaningful to me.

I asked if there were any tests we could run as I listed specific symptoms. I wasn't being hypochondriacal – I was simply being practical.

I wondered if he was listening at all, but he eventually wrote something down and I was encouraged that he might have had an idea. I could clearly see what he had written. He had put at the top of my notes: TATT.

I said, 'What does TATT mean?'

He said, 'It's what we put when someone won't be convinced there's nothing wrong.'

I felt like I'd been slapped in the face. 'You write TATT?'

'Tired all the time,' he said.

I replied, 'Well, I think that shows there is something wrong. Not life-threatening, sure, but someone who is not able to live their life fully. I wouldn't be wasting your time if I just felt a bit tired but could otherwise happily get through each day. I'm not making this up.'

He suddenly lost it with me. 'Oh, for goodness' sake, I just don't know what to do with you. There's nothing else I can do, okay?'

More of a punch than a slap this time.

I ran out in tears.

I hope doctors don't just 'TATT about' still. There are reasons people are ill all the time and exhausted beyond a normal end-of-day tiredness relieved by a night's sleep. TATT means we need help, empathy, a solution. My TATT led to a total collapse, and perhaps it could have been prevented if I had got the diagnosis under that TATT-ery sooner.

Unfortunately, this experience reinforced my unhealthy belief that I couldn't really trust anyone for help. If a professional doctor was going to TATT me about, then I felt stuck. I was officially scared of sharing. And it perpetuated further because without a clear medical diagnosis at this point, I feared ever more I would be misunderstood. If you don't understand the condition you have, how can anyone else? So many of us fear sharing because we don't think people will understand or believe us. Then the more we don't share, the more we all think our secrets are weird.

And with ongoing situations, it's so easy to go quiet. If you're in a tricky marriage, for example, one which you have told a friend about a few times but the problem continues, and you don't want to keep repeating yourself – don't you slowly go quiet? Or if you suffer from anxiety, and you fear being anxious with your friends yet again – don't you hide your feelings? Or if you have a demanding job that wears you down and you can't find a work–life balance, yet you don't feel like you can complain about your toxic workplace any more – don't you keep working?

I think we all just keep going.

And I think it's not just me who at one point couldn't keep

going. Many people hit their own rock-bottoms. Much of this culture of keeping going, of isolation, of loneliness is the root of illness or staying sick, of addiction or toxic relationships. The studies continue to show that longevity of happiness and health – even reducing risk of diabetes and heart disease – is down to safe, meaningful relationships.

It's time to share.

It's time to stop wearing the 'I'm fine' mask.

We're not burdening another by sharing our problems. We're giving them a chance to do what they want to do – to love us.

Stop It!

When I realized sharing (not Cher-ing) in this treasure's context was going against worldy convention in such a strong way, it helped me understand why it was a hard pattern to break. The fear of being rejected means the fear of asking for help. And it's easy to make asking for help complicated when we're unpractised in it.

This is akin to how asking for help initially went for me.

Peers head around the door nervously.

'Ummm, could I just ask . . . actually, don't worry, it's fine . . .'

Scuttles off. Pulls self together. Peers head around door again.

'Umm . . . hi . . . she's back! (wonders why I spoke about myself in the third person) – yes, sorry to disturb, I just wondered . . . actually, don't worry, you're clearly busy, ignore me . . . all fine.'

Runs away. Takes a breath. Says to self, 'Come on, it's worth it, you're doing this to break the cycle for others too . . .'

Prances and sways into the room, trying to be nonchalant and inconspicuous, but looks odd (giraffe like), conspicuous and, indeed, suspicious.

'Hi, sorry (*too loudly*) ME AGAIN! Like a fly to dog poop aren't I – what am I like, such a tit? I wanted to ask for some help with something . . . I mean, if that's okay . . . Don't worry if it's not, do just say . . .'

Gets more anxious as someone responds positively.

'Oh gosh, that's so kind, but seriously, I mean you've got so much on your plate . . .'

Tries to leave but the person remains annoyingly nice and wants to help.

'No, but are you sure, really? You don't actually have to if you don't want . . . Well, let me just tell you what it is . . . just in case . . . Sorry to ask but . . .'

In a roundabout way, with a massive overshare due to panic, (including asking how much wee on sneezing is normal and has anyone else considered padded pants,) asks for some help.

'But really . . . You must say no if you can't. Actually, do you know what, nope . . . It's fine. I'm fine.'

Runs away, picks up burden and carries it away by self again.

Leaves the person trying to help very confused.

Let's just STOP IT, MDRC! I speak for myself. It's so CONFUS-ING and EXHAUSTING! Clarity is kindness. All our posturing to try and be nice and polite and not get in the way is so unclear. I find that when I am unclear, it's not only confusing but often irritating, and indeed often inadvertently unkind. I'm not giving the other person a chance to simply say yes or no – I'm wasting their time, leaving them a little lost or worried.

I needed to stop trapping myself with all this learned cul-tural nonsense. JUST STOP IT MIRANDA!

Unfortunately, that meant accepting and feeling the vul-nerability I didn't realize I needed or indeed I had. Yuck!

To Vulnerability I Go

So disconnected from this part of my inherent identity to belong was I, that I actually thought I had mastered vulnera-bility. I mean, I was good at sharing embarrassing tales socially and indeed even on international chat shows. I burped loudly when I met Jeremy Paxman, not in revolt – I like him – but because one was brewing, and I didn't censor it. And when I met the Queen, I said, 'The pleasure is all yours, ma'am.' (Bit awkward when she didn't realize I was joking.) Turns out that a natural silliness and these kinds of shenanigans are not true vulnerability. It's part of me, sure, but it's not me stripped down to the scared parts and asking for help, feeling my feelings and sharing them.

MDRC, bear with, for I need to share a hard truth of discovery in this treasure – there is absolutely no getting away from understanding and practising vulnerability if you want a truly happy and free life. It's simply not possible. But to encourage you, if it's something you need to work on yourself, I want to tell you something deeply exciting. Drum-roll . . .

I managed it!

I eventually began to clearly say and share what was going on for me and to ask for what I needed. And I jest ye not, I genuinely started to feel a strength, even power, coming into my mind and body when I did. I felt freer, and some energy returning. Yes, energy, even to my TATT-ridden body!

Vulnerability meant I shared some sad family news I received while at work with another person, and had a little weep with her. It opened up the possibility for her to share with me that she was suffering from panic attacks. We are still very close friends.

I asked to hold the hand of a very famous A-list Hollywood star (double vulnerability!) before we walked on-stage, telling him I was nervous because I wasn't feeling very well. I felt so much better in saying it, the nerves almost lifted entirely, and it prompted the other person backstage (otherwise someone who would maintain a high status) to admit he too was nervous, and I then helped him. Sharing vulnerably often frees others. And helping another often reduces fear.

I was happily stopping some of the micro ways I hid and that can affect, amazingly, our health. I mean, get this – I even ask restaurants to turn the music down if I need to, and I would happily ask for food to be taken back if it wasn't hot enough (I'm almost not British any more . . .).

As it dawned on me that I'd become isolated because I didn't previously understand how to be vulnerable, I was looking forward to busting the myth once and for all of it feeling safer to go it alone or 'get it together'. To see that not allowing ourselves any weakness – whether that's a simple tiredness, a common cold, a difficult day at work, an emotional reaction, a problem we have let grow and now feel shame about, let alone more acute illness or difficulty – is just downright mean and stressful. It makes life hard and scary for ourselves.

Of course we're allowed to be weak. In fact, weak is not the right word. It has such negative connotations even though it simply means not having the resources for a moment to do something. I think exposed is a good word because it's how we all are (metaphorically – please don't be cheeky, MDRC). We're human beings exposed to a difficult world; of course we all have times of 'weakness' when we need people and help. Nobody is invincible. But that is one of the masks we try and wear (or have been led to believe we need to wear if we want to 'get ahead'). We're designed to negotiate our amazing, incredible, surprising lives that will inevitably come with trials by connecting to ourselves and to others. Admitting we are vulnerable when we are is such a relief. More to the point: being vulnerable is by far the strongest stance to take. A superpower. What a relief, and how dare the world have told us otherwise? We don't have to have it all sorted.

We are all vulnerable in different ways. Let's not forget that some people are exposed and feel at risk just by nature of who they are, be it their gender, race or sexuality. Others might need financial support. Some lack energetic resources and need day-to-day tasks done for them (hands up). Some need help with their relationships. Some with their sense of self-worth. Some need administrative help with their workload. We all need help. It's our vulnerability that connects us.

It's easy to spout now. It did take me some time. I was fiercely independent, practical and goal-orientated, therefore being debilitated by illness was a massive assault on how I'd been living. I had been the strong one. I could work long hours. I was professionally and socially confident. I was also often the wise one and, ironically, would be asked for and happily give advice. But being unwell made me realize I was also fiercely independent in a negative way – not needing people, having a fear of being weak, buttressing with an armour of self-confidence and self-belief. Some of those traits I feel lucky to have. But many of them I've slowly chipped away at, and I do things joyously differently. That is, I'm still confident and hopefully wise at times, but I now accept that I'm also always going to be vulnerable and need people. I am more honest, and it's such a blooming relief.

'You can be vulnerable and still be powerful. You can have a gentle heart, but still be rock-solid at your core. You can be gentle as a breeze, but as fierce as a dragon. The best people always embody both sides.' – Author unknown

If we just show our strong or silly sides, we're only developing friendships on one level. If we show our friends every aspect, then we're developing true, healing connection. It's easy to feel lonely even among friends when we haven't dared to be honest with them.

But, MDRC, choose your people wisely (or person – we don't have to share with everyone). Ultimately our mind and body are looking for that feeling of safety and dignity when we share with another. And, if sharing openly with people you know feels like too big a step for you, then think of other ways you can connect that make you feel safe. I found that an intentional cuddle or a look in Peggy's eyes would give me a felt sense of love. (Where would we be without animals? To remind you, Peggy is a dog ... It might have sounded like I was cuddling a random old lady ...)

All I can say is, when I allowed myself to share some difficult times, I noticed how much deeper and stronger my friendships went.

No more brave-faced masks for me.

Seriously, Stop It!

I once spent a weekend with a few friends, and a week later one of them said, 'Oh, I wish we'd gone on a walk while we were there.' I replied, 'But I asked if you wanted to go on one and you said no,' and they said, 'I didn't think you wanted to go so I said no.' Can we just all STOP IT?!

The very English conversation had gone like this:

Her: What a lovely day.
Me: Yes, shall we go for a walk?
Her: Oh yes, maybe, that would be lovely.
Me: Great, well, let me know.
A couple of hours later.
Me: How are you feeling about that walk?
Her: I'd be happy to go if you want to.
Me: Well, no, only if you want to.
Her: Well, don't go for me. Only if you want to.
Me: No, I do want to go, but only if you want to go.
Her: Are you sure you want to go? You don't have to.
Me (feeling confused – clarity is kindness!): Do you
*   want to go for a walk?*
Her: Well, it's a lovely day.
Me: Yes, but do you want to go for a walk?
Her: There's no need to go for a walk just for me.
Me: I'd like to go if you want to go.
Her: No, honestly, don't worry, let's leave it. I'll put the
*   kettle on.*
Me: Okay.

I was longing to go but wanted her to be clear what she wanted, and she was longing to go but was too scared to say what she wanted and read in that I didn't want to go. We sat inside quietly having a cup of tea, looking outside, longing to be walking and chatting as we did.

It makes me sad when we miss out on even the tiniest opportunity that could be a moment we may never forget, or that's just plain lovely and fun and a way to connect better.

Dare to state a want.

Dare to share.

And dare to share if you want to listen to Cher. Sorry . . . (also not sorry).

A Tree Blooms For Help

The ongoing paradox in this and further treasures is that what keeps us at our wild, natural, best selves is usually the opposite to what the world has conditioned many of us to do and feel.

When a glorious, wild tree is ailing in any way – perhaps it has a fungus or lacks some vital nutrient – it asks for help. All trees are interconnected under the forest floor and support each other (fascinating documentaries out there if you are so inclined, such as the wonderful *Trees and Other Entanglements*). And one way a tree asks for help is it blooms early in the season. An untrained eye might assume it's healthy and strong for blooming before others. Actually, it's boldly and beautifully signalling a weakness. It's gathering nutrients while it can, hoping for more time to spread its seed to extend its cycle of life, and sending a signal to the trees around it that it will need support to survive.

That tree holds no shame for having a moment of attack, illness, difficulty, 'weakness'. It simply knows that to ask for help is the natural order of things, and because it knows it's worthy of it. By just existing, it is worthy.

That's wildness right there.

Those who are able to be vulnerable believe they are worthy. With that belief, they are safe to seek love without fear of rejection. They're asking for help, rightly, because they know they matter.

Bloom like a tree to ask for help when you need it. We want to love you. You matter, MDRC.

Listen Up

There's one big issue about sharing I discovered and can't ignore in our first treasure. And that is this: a culture not taught to be vulnerable means a culture not always good at listening.

For starters, when listening we can go into fixing mode. I was a terrible fixer – loved going straight to the advice. But being fixed is not what we need when we're sharing. My research taught me that it is in fact often harmful. It can reinforce the alleged fear that we are inherently bad and need sorting out. I found it incredibly interesting and useful to discover that if someone is trying to fix another person, saying it will all be fine, or invalidating their story, it's usually because they have invalidated their own and aren't ready to confront the difficulty within them, whether they know it or not. Trying to fix someone is not helpful or kind unless that person is asking for specific advice. It's a quick solution that can communicate that we don't have time for the other.

What we need, which is why therapy can be so invaluable, is to be listened to non-judgementally. The fear of our situation can lessen when we see that experience being held in gentleness and kindness by another. There's an extraordinary man called Gregory Boyle who set up Homeboy Industries in Los Angeles, which is now the world's largest gang intervention and rehabilitation programme (let's never forget how much good there is out there), and he says:

'It would seem that, quite possibly, the ultimate measure of health in any community might well reside in our ability to stand in awe at what folks have to carry rather than in judgement at how they carry it.'

Wow, beautiful.

It's always going to be worth sitting with our own awkwardness as we listen to another bravely sharing. They'll likely be feeling awkward too. There we find that clear and authentic relationship. We may fear it, but intrinsically we love getting to know each other. As another good man, Mister Rogers said:

'To love someone is to strive to accept that person exactly the way that he or she is, right there and now.'

Gathering Onwards

Even in the midst of the darkness of illness, I became truly excited about the idea of rekindling friendships. I knew my natural, wild self was healthy when I was being vulnerable and honest with chosen close friends. Just the idea of that and I felt closer to the concept of coming home to myself. Genuinely, I would have traded in any past success for true connection. I had experienced how aloneness can be severley detrimental to the body.

I admitted again that I was longing for love within a romantic relationship too, for that one person who truly got me, but my hope for that was very, very slim. I had Peggy for now. My dog husband!

And I knew the most important thing was to keep exploring the treasures I might learn on this journey through the cave. There would be no point learning how to share and connect better if I was still suffering from a degree of fatigue and a compromised immune system that made gatherings and parties impossible. I still had to find answers for my health.

But it was exciting in the moment just to want to socialize in that wider way again. I have always had a passion for socializing in free, authentic, fun ways. In rather divine timing, I happened upon an episode of a podcast on 'the art of gathering'. It helped me see that in addition to losing the art of listening, we've also lost the understanding of what it truly is to gather. A gathering means an assembly or meeting, especially one held for a specific purpose. That being the key – a purpose. For an event to captivate us and make us feel joyful and present to the occasion, there needs to be a clear intention behind it. Yet I believe so many people hold or attend social events from that hidden, masked place of needing to be approved. I've noticed people saying they 'should' attend because it would be rude not to, or feeling they needed to be seen there, or were rushing, knowing it was one thing too many in the diary, but on the make-up and fake smiles would go to brave the night out. Because, you know, 'We should, shouldn't we?' No, we shouldn't, I say. Not like that.

When we gather for a reason, we can love and be of service, and we're excited to be there.

How many times have you been polite and kind just to be polite and kind? When a friend told me she had to get off the phone because she was heading to a party, I said, 'Ooh, lovely, have fun.' She replied that she was dreading it. It was her neighbours' party, so she thought she'd just sneak in, make her face known and leave as soon as possible. I got quite cross! Turned into a bit of a headmistress. 'How would you like it if someone came to your party in dread and then snuck away as soon as possible? You're being rude and insensitive.' She defended herself understandably by saying she didn't want to be rude by saying no. I suggested that she was being far ruder by going and leaving early when they'd gone to such effort and might worry that she wasn't enjoying it. Plus she was getting up really early the next morning for a long day and she'd told me how much she was needing a rest. I pointed out she was lying to herself too. She was being polite and kind to be polite and kind, which meant she wasn't being polite and kind. We abandon our needs as well as that of our friends by turning up dishonourably. I truly believe that if we knew someone was coming to meet us in those circumstances, we would be deeply offended.

Unless we're turning up to gather with love, having carved out that time for clear purpose, then we are not there honourably. For me it's back to 'clarity is kindness'. We mistake masks and politeness for kindness. I don't think they are. Let's turn up honourably, authentically, or not at all. Hark at me!

I heard a story of a woman bored by the endless small talk at the coffee mornings she attended with her school mum friends. She decided to be brave and suggest that they turn their meetings into 'tea and tantrum' gatherings, because she was feeling so fed up and tired and needed to vent. Everyone was so relieved and attendance soared with energy and glee. They loved the chance to be real, and their moaning naturally led to much laughter and healing. They broke the polite sheen of convention as they gathered for a reason. I love that!

I'm now very specific about any hosting I do. To the extent that every time I have anything resembling a party (I say party – it's usually max ten friends and a dress code of pyjamas), I provide a timetable of the event. Everyone likes to relax within a structure! It's easy to do when you host specifically – I might have people over to watch something (*Strictly*

Come Dancing being the natural example, or a fun film, definitely sporting events), or I might gather for a sing-along (a yearly event minimum for a group of us at Christmas), or for a celebration, a catch-up to encourage a friend, or a crafts session! And a timetable means I'm super relaxed hosting because, for example, I've said before people arrive that I want them out by 9.30 pm so I can go to bed. Such freedom. At 9.25 pm, if they're looking too comfortable, I start shouting, 'Open the Uber app, please!' A friend of mine plays 'Climb Ev'ry Mountain' very loudly when she's hit a wall of overwhelm and wants people to leave. They know she's serious and they all have a massive sing-along as they head to the door. Genius!

Surely, we'd all much rather connect with each other when we know why and how much we are helping? The vulnerability to gather for specific reasons becomes joyful for all.

Are you galvanized to gather with me for Treasure Two, MDRC? I hope so, because although gathering and sharing are so often about pure fun, the next treasure happens to be my ickiest as I faced my illness head-on. Don't worry, all shall be well – it also turned out to have a nugget of wisdom in helping me move towards safely connecting again. Go treasures!

Let's fortify with a dance break. It would be rude to end this treasure without doing some Cher-ing . . . I'm off to Shoop Shoop again . . .

Treasure Two

Surrender

TREASURES PICKED UP: Surrender, trust, hope, acceptance, stillness, vulnerability is strength

PATTERNS SMASHED: Overriding, pushing, fixing, avoiding, over-independence

WATCHWORD: Faithfulness

SOUNDTRACK: 'In the Waiting' by Kina Grannis

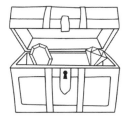

Surrender

Wasps vs Picnics

So, I had become energized about sharing, connecting and gathering. I was on the new, exciting path to free that wild self and forge ahead. And then I was hit with the next treasure: learning how to surrender. Surrender? Umm. Doesn't sound very rousing. To put it mildly.

To be honest with you, MDRC, the early part of the cave does get a little murky. But the concept of surrender surprised me in becoming – truly – the surefire foundation to a calm, healthy life. It was vital for my health condition but applies to many a difficult situation. I so hope I can explain it clearly enough, for I did find it the hardest treasure to get to grips with. But it became the bedrock of my life and led to the lighter, more fun treasures ahead.

Let me use a light explanation initially. I think we can split people into two groups: those who serenely settle into a pose of surrender and acceptance in challenging moments, and those who fight and flee (my hand is firmly raised!). Now, imagine yourself settling down to an idyllic picnic. You've opened the Tupperware of mini Scotch eggs (you're only human), a lovely MOIST cucumber sandwich is in hand, and you can't wait to get to the scones. Everything is glorious. And then – a pesky wasp descends.

At this point, there are two ways to react. There is the person who remains in sandwich-eating position and waves the wasp gently away, trusting they are unlikely to sting and will eventually leave, and won't let it ruin their otherwise beautiful picnic. The other type of person (my hand has shot up again) will get instantly irritated – and possibly anxious – by the sight or sound of said wasp. They will start doing a, what I call, panic waft, desperately trying to get it away because, frankly, everything was perfect and now look – all is ruined, typical! If a second wasp appears, this person perceives sudden and severe danger and is up on their feet running from the beasts, screeching, battling an invisible monster with a napkin (the wasps long flew in the other direction). No one can understand what they are doing – perhaps it's a strange dance routine or they've just lost the plot with life for a moment. As the sweaty napkin-waving-panic-wafter returns, the calm-carry-on-picnicking person has finished their sandwich, popped a couple of Scotch eggs, and is joyfully plunging into their scone because they have simply put a jam jar strategically *away* from the rug so that any wasps head in its direction.

How do they do it?!

Once, a wasp got too close to my cleavage and I assumed it had dived down (well, it's excellent cleavage) to sting me violently on the nipple (imagine) or get lodged in another part of my clothing. It was so alarming a thought, I lost any moral or social compass and very quickly removed all my clothes to avert crisis. The panic-wafter now upgraded to panic-stripper. One slight issue – to my fellow picnickers, I simply looked like I was choosing to strip for them, for they hadn't identified there was a wasp in the equation. They stared. I curtsied – it seemed the right next step.

Suffice to say, the non-panic-wafting, non-screaming, non-stripping soul has accepted that we live in a world with wasps that sometimes attend our picnics. They have had a lovely time saving energy by neither panicking nor being angry with the situation.

I am not wired with this particular life skill. I lack the inherent trust that things will just 'work out'. When I collapsed with illness and was unable to crack on with life through natural fighting spirit alone, I floundered. I tried to resist the wasp. I wanted, with every fibre of my being, to fight against, rather than to face, my reality. That's what we do, that's wild, isn't it – to fight and fix and force on?

Well, MDRC, it turns out that neuroscience says, 'What you resist persists.' Sorry, what? I didn't like the sound of that.

The mindfulness experts Mark Williams and Danny Penman say in their book, *Mindfulness: Finding Peace in a Frantic World*, 'It's often far easier and more effective in the long run to live with our difficulties than to pour resources into battling and suppressing them.' Is it though? No, I still didn't like this idea at all, MDRC. I preferred the idea that I could push difficulties firmly away and not face them! But the scientists kept piping up with that annoying little phrase, 'What you resist persists.'

What fresh hell is this?! Into the murky part of the cave I had to go.

'There's Nothing Wrong Here Right Now'

As I continued to study the 'ists' on this matter, another phrase stood out: 'There's nothing wrong here right now.' WHAT?! It seemed not only implausible but downright mean. Frankly, I would have punched someone in the face had they coolly said this to me when I was collapsed with exhaustion. I would have shouted, 'Um, excuse me, but EVERYTHING is wrong! I can't get out of bed, I'm alone, no one understands, my dreams and hopes for my life are fading away, nothing is right right now, it's wrong and that's why it's all so blooming awful. I am all full of wrong, so – and I mean this with no respect at all – GO AWAY, THANK YOU TO YOU!'

Turns out, what the phrase actually means is accepting what *is*. The clever 'ists' are saying that despite being in a situation you would assuredly not choose, if there is nothing you can do about it at that moment, then there is no choice but to accept it is happening. And if you stop focusing solely on what is wrong – on the wasp – there might be ways to make it manageable. Because at the very least, you are already living it. Like a true warrior. Many of us in difficult times say, 'I can't do this,' or, 'This is unbearable,' yet we are doing it. I'm welling up thinking of the myriad stories of people hit with ghastly events but who heroically keep taking the next breath. Please applaud yourself and whatever you feel like a warrior about right now.

The 'ists' even suggested it's possible to get to, 'Okay, this is what is meant to be happening in this moment, so I can accept and live it.' I mean, that's ninja-level supernatural calm-ery and I'm still amazed when I get anywhere close to it. All I know for sure is that through acceptance, a lot of suffering can be eased. Or rather, suffering about the suffering. I knew that physical and emotional pain, darkness of all kinds, was an uncontrollable part of life, and now came the notion that much of that pain is actually caused by the resistance to pain, focusing on pain, fear of the pain, judging the pain.

They were not telling me to deny my situation and illness, but instead saying that if I confronted it compassionately – instead of furiously wanting it to go away – perhaps I could bend towards finding a way to accept it. The alternative wasn't working – every time I wished my symptoms to be different, every time I protested being bed- or housebound, I was only adding fuel to an already stressful situation. Frightening myself. Like I was constantly watching a bad news reel.

Okay, yes, I concede, the theory makes sense. Breathe, and have a look around for some sliding cats instead.

In retrospect, I can see how exhausting it was to try to wish away an illness. To be constantly fighting reality is, as speaker and author Byron Katie says, akin to spending your life trying to teach a cat to bark. I was living it, so it would be kinder to accept it. Because we can't cultivate more than there is in this moment. There is so much we can only surrender to. We can't slow time. We can't make the countryside different. We can't change people. We can't stop the ageing process (not even by changing our faces). We can't change the weather, or the TV schedules, or the suffering, or where we were born, or what our natural skills are. And that is okay because that is how it is.

After a few weeks – no, I will be honest, months – of berating and not accepting my weak body, I dared to keep reading about this whole surrender and acceptance malarkey. One day I read: 'Surrender is not about giving up. But it is also not doing this: I am fine, push on, ignore what the body is saying, keep going, I can overcome this.' It *finally* clicked that not allowing ourselves to be who and how we are is dishonest and therefore exhausting and terrifying.

I began to understand it all more intellectually. I read more fantastic, life-giving quotes like this one from Dorothy Hunt's poem 'Peace Is This Moment Without Judgment':

Peace is this moment without thinking
that it should be some other way,
that you should feel some other thing,
that your life should unfold according to your plans.

Peace is this moment without judgement,
this moment in the Heart-space where
everything that is is welcome.

Yes, lovely, calming. But, for me at the time, it was only calming for a very brief moment. This whole concept was still completely new to me. It was still only theory, so all that came tumbling out was: 'I WANT TO BE BETTER AND FOR

74

MY LIFE TO UNFOLD ACCORDING TO ALL MY PLANS! HOW DO YOU DO IT?! I don't want to be sick. How is this moment peaceful?! I'M NOT GOING TO SURRENDER! I want to be fit and functioning. Sorry, 'ists', you are probably all wrong in the face.'

I couldn't do it. I didn't want to face my reality. Or I wasn't ready.

It was easier because it was all I knew, to keep distracting and keep fighting. I wondered if I had always been like this – a natural fighter, a fleer, a panic-wafter (and sometimes-stripper) – or if my current circumstances were made scarier by the lack of diagnosis and scarring past TATT-ery.

The Twisted Ankle

I remember the time I was skipping excitedly into the BBC for a *Comic Relief* rehearsal – the show was going live on TV that night, and while I was always thrilled heading into the BBC, live TV and *Comic Relief* added to the excitement. I was presenting with David Walliams and we'd been rehearsing a dance for our set (two more elegant dancers you are VERY likely to meet). I wasn't literally skipping in, but I might as well have been as I tripped on a rocky bit of pavement. On trying to steady myself, I landed on the edge of a pothole and was soon on the ground writhing in the horrid pain that is going over on your ankle. Both luckily and embarrassingly, someone was passing by. They helped me up and I hobbled into a dressing room. I lay on a tiny two-seater sofa with my feet dangling over the edge (I hope it was a tiny sofa as it made me feel like a giant), ankle throbbing.

What I should have done in my best interest, had I the emotional agility, was surrender to and accept this temporary situation: *I have a twisted ankle. Hey ho. What can I possibly do about it apart from lie here and wait for the answers to unfold?*

Instead, what I did in a very mature way was screech, 'Well, this is blooming TYPICAL, isn't it? I won't be able to perform now, and I've worked really hard on this and really, really wanted to do it. Why do these things always happen to ME? And, and . . . I was getting fit, and I won't be able to keep exercising now, life is sooooo disappointing . . .' Down that merry self-pitying thought tunnel I went.

The reality was that in that moment, I was as comfortable as my long body could be on a miniature sofa. I was alive, breathing and being looked after. Nonetheless, I chose full-on grumpiness! Embracing the additional 'I'm letting everyone down' stress, as if it was my fault I'd gone over on my ankle. Completely wasted energy, MDRC, because I embarrassingly admit it really was okay – I *was* able to perform (albeit with heavy ankle strapping and pain), eventually I started exercising again and Nothing Major Happened. I could have avoided so much stress, adrenalin and negative energy by surrendering and accepting 'it is what it is'.

Yup, it's official, I have always been a bit of a panic-wafter! I wasn't going to berate myself because most humans instinctively rile against difficulty and attempt to stay in control. But trying to control life is anxious behaviour. I had no idea how much I had been scaring myself by trying to control things that I could never influence. There were big changes I wanted and needed to make going forward, but progess is of course about learning the changes we can make and surrendering to the ones we can't.

Reflecting back on my petulant response to the ankle, I knew one major thing I wanted to change was my negative reaction to things that I didn't like or didn't think should be happening. I did want to move towards acceptance and sur-render. But, I admit, at the time, it still felt too hard. If I was like that with a twisted ankle, just imagine when I ended up bed-bound for years. I riled like the best of them. I was expert at riling!

If I heard, 'This too shall pass,' I'd instinctively whisper, 'Oh, do shut up!'

If I read, 'The way you feel now is not the way you will always feel,' I would sigh and say, 'Oh, now you "ists" are just saying the same thing in different fancy ways.' (I was, of course, talking to a book.)

This was the worst: 'Bloom where you've been planted.' I replied: 'Oh no, now please do shut up once and for all. I blooming well can't bloom, thank you very much. I'm far from blooming – I barely feel like a seed, let alone a bulb that might bloom – so stop telling me I can blooming well bloom right now, for I feel wholly bloom-less. This is a bloom-free zone!'

So, Why Is It So Hard?

I mean seriously, surrendering is obviously true and wise and healing and the way to make life easier, so why did I find it quite so hard? On talking to some friends and family, I discovered I wasn't the only one, so I was determined to find the patterns we might be in that make it distinctly tough. I discovered two key reasons.

The first: the world has been shouting the opposite at us. And let me take this opportunity to remind you what I mean by 'the world'. I mean the contemporary culture, the rules, practices and trends we have been led to believe are true. In this instance, the shouts that say: keep going, never give in, push, push, push, do, do, do, achieve, go, go, go. As adults, the busier you are, the supposedly 'cooler' and 'better' you are – produce, enjoy, be happy, party, accrue. I for one came to believe that was the wild, natural way to live life to the full. I wasn't a workaholic, but I was certainly a productivity junkie. Even on holiday I would make sure I was maxing the shit out of the day (sorry to do another shit at you, as it were) – had I done enough, seen enough, what about that sunset boat trip, should I do that? I was ruining holidays with 'achievement' – like a terrifying holiday rep pacing and shouting at people on a sun lounger: 'Come on, are you doing this fun as well as you can? Are you making sure you're having the BEST FUN EVER?!' It makes me think of the quote, 'If we'd stop trying to be happy, we could have a pretty good time.'

There is hard-wiring in many of us to focus on the aim to just be happy: WE WANT IT ALL AND WE WANT IT NOW!

78

I also love the quote by philosopher Eric Hoffer: 'The search for happiness is one of the chief sources of unhappiness.' Feelings of 'I want it sorted and to be well NOW' and 'I just want to be happy' came up for me time after time. Exhausting. Of course there would be relief in relinquishing control. Of course there would be relief if my aim was to face what was happening in my life as best I could, rather than focusing on any lack with the quest to be happy.

THE WORLD SAYS *fight, battle, push, fix, control, achieve, override, get out of the way of your feelings to keep doing, constant achievement should be applauded, vulnerability is weakness so hide your anxiety, stay upbeat and positive, striving is rock-solid healthy living, listening to your feelings and issues is a waste of time and selfish namby-pamby nonsense. Happiness is your goal. Success makes you a good person.*

It seemed a much wiser option to adhere to the new way that was being gently whispered to me in the dark cave.

THE TRUTH SAYS *the way to peace and healing is acceptance, trust, hope, self-compassion and rest. Vulnerability is strength, and surrender is a place of transformation, a courageous place from which to say 'help'. We are designed as emotional beings. Life is up and down, darkness is allowed, and trials are often great teachers and part of living life to the full. Meaningful work is wonderful if you get it, but what you achieve is not who you are.*

I so wanted to move from theory to practice, to turn away from my conditioned culture and become accepting of where

I was at and listen to what was needed for me to recover and get stronger. Why did it remain so hard?

This led me to the second reason. If surrender means learning how to be still with 'what is', then that means we might have to feel some – wait for it – EMOTIONS. Even the notion! I mean, I could portray feelings as an actor, but in the real life with my friends and family? Yuck! That really takes the biscuit! (And often leads me to literally taking the biscuit. Eating your feelings, anyone?) Sitting with uncomfortable thoughts and feelings is something we are not taught to do. All the masks of fear, fighting, fixing, busyness and productivity have also been used to hide the feelings and experiences we don't feel we should be having or showing. NO WONDER WE'RE ALL SO KNACKERED! But unless we surrender and accept, we can't change a circumstance. Or cope with a circumstance. We can't operate from a place of strength that is admitting vulnerability and asking for help. Instead, it's all too easy to self-criticize and judge what's happening to us. When you think about it, that's just mean!

Fighting and trying to fix my situation, I realized, ultimately meant wanting my life and my very self to be 'better' – some mythical best self that was better than the real me now. So mean! The pressure to be anything other than who we are can only ever be scary and stressful. It's not a dignified or safe way to treat ourselves, and our nervous system will react accordingly.

So here I was, learning to tune out the shouting world and getting on to the new surrendered frequency. Deep down, a frequency I knew to be true. But. The world's voice IS SO

LOUD. It's very, very hard to get out of the mindset that our parents, their parents, our teachers, schools, jobs, other people and anything and anyone in the world (ultimately industrialization and capitalism, if we're really facing it all head-on) have been shouting at us – that we must only ever soldier on, and that to keep doing, producing, achieving is strong and noble and admirable.

I was in that place. It was wholly ingrained. I had always lived by, 'I'm a strong independent woman, I can sort it.' It was inbuilt in me like a stick of rock that productivity was the way to happiness. Over and over again I drowned out the new kind voice, and I carried on carrying on.

Brace, Brace, Brace

On a hot day in May, the first really hot day since my collapse, I felt strong enough to lie in the sun for a bit. I lay on my stomach and heard one of those kindly wise internal whispers say, 'Let the sun melt your muscles into the earth to take your weight.' As I breathed a sigh of release, it was clear how tense I was. The kindly voice continued, 'Can you let the warmth on your back feel like an infusion of love, a love for just being you, just lying there, nothing to prove?'

I knew more than ever, in that moment, that this productivity junkie needed to find rest. I was mainly still fighting against my situation because I thought if I gave in to how I felt I would drown in it all (I didn't yet have the tools to face feeling what I was feeling), and I would never be able to get back to work and all I wanted to do. I kept looking for answers, trying new supplements or exercises, assessing the symptoms and therefore giving them power over me and noticing and fearing every twinge. But staying upset and fighting so hard only keeps our bodies braced and alert – which is *not* what a sick body needs to heal. If you are bracing, your breath is shallower, muscles tighter; you are restless and likely have a whirring negative mind causing sleeplessness too. I noticed a lovely loop emerged: when I felt sensations I didn't want, like fatigue, I tried to override them, which activated muscles to fight, which made me feel more fatigued, which got me more annoyed, which risked leading to a secondary condition like a bad back or gut issues – and on the unhelpful carrying on carrying on loop goes.

I lay there, feeling the sun on my back, letting it be medicine. An IV of love. Could I slow down and tune out the world's shouts? Could I really face how I was feeling? My body released another sigh at the idea. As I came to learn, not striving to be any other way than how you are with what's going on in that moment is incredibly nourishing and healing. I knew my mind and body couldn't heal with the current level of resistance. Was my initial hunch right that these treasures might show me a new way to do life, which meant my body could get healthy? Was this moment, however fleeting, the start of me facing my vulnerabilities within my illness however scary it felt?

It turns out I had one big lesson left to learn on surrender. Stick with my murkiness, MDRC, for the lesson was a big, heavy revvy (that's a lovely way a friend calls a heavy revelation, which I have adopted).

Facing The Monster

The biggest reason we find it hard to surrender to a situation that's causing us pain is 'simply' because we're scared or terrified of that situation. Of course we are – that's why it's causing us the pain and angst that it is. If we're terrified of something, we'll naturally fight it and run away from it. Of course we do! It's the current enemy of our life – our wasp, our monster – and we want to be free of it. My monster was being trapped by confusing, and frightening, symptoms of illness (particularly so whilst still waiting for a clarity of diagnosis). For others it might be anxiety, burn-out, a phobia, chronic tension, discontentment, not believing you are loved for who you are. (The list could be endless, sadly.)

I had to face that the research was not only right but the way forward – what you resist persists, and if you turn to 'face the monster', it will lessen. It seems SO counter-intuitive. Such a challenging concept. To that end, the clinician that I learnt from – a marvellous 'ist' by the name of John Gasienica – has put it in his words to help. (And I feel it my duty to say that if you're suffering from chronic pain, then his colleague Alan Gordon has written a book, *The Way Out*, which has helped or healed many.)

Now concentrate, MDRC, this is the therapy-ish bit! But from where all the good stuff can come . . .

Our brain is constantly trying to predict whether things around us are safe or dangerous. When we avoid something, we're encouraging our brain to predict that thing is dangerous. If we avoid it enough, our brain begins to label it as catastrophic and activates a full-blown fear response whenever we encounter it.

Okay, yup, makes sense, John. It would be like me shouting at a sweet, young child with my symptoms: 'Yes, you should be scared, this situation is AWFUL, these symptoms and feelings are ALL WRONG, oh my God, did you feel that?, be very scared, maybe we should go to hospital, OH MY GOD, is that a wasp, RUN!' We wouldn't do that. We would sit down next to a scared child, hold them and say, 'It's okay, I'm here,' and the child would naturally be in the present moment with less fear.

John goes on (we love John) . . .

The best way to change our brain's danger prediction is to go towards the thing we're afraid of – to intentionally get exposure to it. If you're afraid of dogs, you can read all the statistics that show how safe dogs are. But until you actually spend time with a nice dog who harmlessly sits on your lap, you won't completely get over your fear. When you interact with something you once feared and come away from the experience feeling safer, that's called a corrective experience.

Okay, a bit more challenging, John, but yes . . . I'm with you . . . I don't want to be afraid of what I'm experiencing.

When we continue to expose ourselves to the thing we fear and have corrective experiences, our brain begins to shed the 'dangerous' label altogether, and no longer activates a fear response. It often means asking people to sacrifice comfort in the short term so that they can feel safe in the long term. This is not an easy sell, but often necessary for recovery.

It's definitely not an easy sell, John. But we still love you. And it makes complete sense. That braced position comes from the brain's fear response, and if I could sit with and allow my symptoms (however grim they may feel), then the fear response would go away and in turn the symptoms would lessen. By running away from something, I was not instilling in myself a sense of strength and resilience that I could cope with the situation. Or a trust that the circumstance could change.

As lovely John says, it's uncomfortable a notion to turn around and face the monster – NO SHIT, SHERLOCK! – and that's why we all just carry on carrying on.

Something exciting clicked as regards the first two treasures. This feels obvious now but was a real aha moment. A great nugget! I realized that it's no wonder when we're asked how we are, we so easily say, 'Yeah, fine, thanks, I'm good,' when we're not. How can we share if we haven't faced and accepted where we are at ourselves? Or if we're in shame about what we are experiencing or how we are behaving. (As an aside: I think it's so important to give ourselves enormous lumps of grace, even if we can't do what we know we need to do. It takes us as long as it takes us.) My aha moment meant I was more incentivized to surrender. I know scientifically now that when I say I'm fine when I am not, I end up subconsciously more braced. If I'm not being honest with myself, then I can but just carry on carrying on.

I was grateful to finally side with the 'ists'. I was surrendering to the idea of surrender.

Crashed Again, But It Came Good

Plus, if I am honest, I was given no choice. MDRC, my dear body finally got my attention – after an attempt to go back to work – by crashing (significantly) again. Yup, I took one for the team to prove soldiering on truly doesn't work!

I was pretty much bed-bound again for another few months. Fatigue is very hard to describe, especially as everyone occasionally suffers from tiredness. But this was back to that total ghost-like weakness. Eventually I was moving about a bit, but a walk outside was as hard as anything I had done. I would stand still in the road feeling as if I had to remind my brain how to put one foot in front of the other. I would look at a cup of tea on the table and wonder if I had the strength to take a sip.

I really hated being forced to look at this monster. I absolutely loved my work, and knowing I couldn't continue with it was one of many things that was heart-wrenching for me. I remember hearing that kind and wise voice within: 'Who is to say that this isn't part of your story, that good can't come from this? It's not honest to try and keep shining bright when your light has gone out.' I was so ready to get angry and say, 'Oh, do shut up,' as per, but I didn't get sucked in (progress) and focused on the day's only task ahead of me: to take dear Peggy around the block for a little walk. And in doing so, I did learn something good.

I was shuffling along the street in my fog of fatigue when I bumped into the local dog walker and her pack of hounds.

Peggy started yapping, a little afraid of the other dogs suddenly confronting her. I wasn't really concentrating and instinctively tried to drag myself and Peggy away. The dog walker then said something to me that still smarts.

'Your poor dog,' she said. I looked at her, confused. 'You need to reassure her, be top dog, teach her to follow you, not drag her, or let her run ahead.'

The stress was instantaneous, so I mumbled an 'Okay, thanks,' and slowly moved off. But she continued, 'We used to laugh at you, in the park. You were so often on your phone and not paying any attention to your dog. I mean, what is the point in having a dog if you don't play with them and give them the attention they need?'

I was shocked and biting my lip not to cry. She was projecting her own assumptions on to me that were nowhere near the truth. She had no idea that Peggy was my rock and best friend during a very isolated time of my life, that I was weak and confused, and desperate to get back home before I couldn't walk any further. She saw someone tall, strong and successful in that moment. Not untrue. But she didn't see the fragile, weepy human underneath. The good I learnt in that moment is that we never know what's going on for anyone – we all carry a lot, even if we're pretending we're fine. (That dear dog walker herself might have just had the worst day of her life for all I knew.)

Further good came on realizing the pain of the misunderstanding from this woman was the same pain I was giving myself by not accepting my situation. We, in effect, ignore, shame, misunderstand and don't listen to ourselves. Pushing on is not kindly. I wasn't going to fight any more. No more carrying on carrying on for me.

What's The Next Right Action?

As I first turned towards surrender, there was a bit of bumpy air (not just my personal wind – IBS was a secondary issue . . . what do you mean I'm oversharing?) due to facing all those feelings and needs for the first time.

In fact, brace yourselves – oops, wrong choice of word, *don't* brace yourselves as that's bad for your body and brain – calmly accept what I'm about to say. I know that many of us like to avoid our feelings or see them as a monster. Such doers are we, we've come to believe that meeting our emotional needs is just an added extra if we're lucky to find the time. Bless us. But Treasure Three will be about how to feel our feelings.

It's important to go there because ignoring ourselves and our needs is another disaster to good health. None of us would sit back and let an infected wound on our skin fester. You wouldn't look at the blisters and pus and reddening and just go, 'Oh gosh, that's so annoying, I have too much to do, I will just bung a plaster on it and crack on.' No, you would know that soon enough you would be in deep pain and a very medically serious situation. Well, it's EXACTLY THE SAME with conditions that are not externally present on our bodies: burn-out, anxiety, chronic pain, not to mention situations that are heartbreaking and emotionally hard. When you think about it this way, isn't it madness that we so often ignore what we are feeling and going through?

But one step at a time. I remembered a good tip from an 'ist' (I was not shouting at them any more) which simply said, 'Ask yourself: what's the next right action in the now to move forward?' Instead of angrily berating and avoiding, what is the kindly next right action I can take now I'm accepting my reality? It could be finding a trusted friend to confide in or eating crisps in the bath. The question gives space to consider the specific things we may need help with. Each next right action breeds confidence and resilience as we take the positive steps we can to move ahead, which in turn creates a clearer head to make the next right step and the next. As Einstein said, 'We can't solve problems with the same thinking that created them.' It's a great hack because very rarely do we think a kind right next action is to PANIC! Nor is it, 'I know, I think I'll ignore how I am feeling and be really angry with what's happening and blame everyone around me, including myself.'

For me the next right action was, and still often is, having a cup of tea or sometimes a snack. Correction: it's always having a cup of tea and a snack . . . And in the many weeks and months after the second collapse, it was simply sitting at the window to absorb nature (with a cup of tea and a snack). I had a rare opportunity in conceding to this confinement to watch the seasons. And it was settling, MDRC. I watched the weather changing, the clouds, the leaves, to remind myself that the one assurance we have is that things *always* change. It helped remind me when I 'faced the monster' aka my symptoms, that they too would change, naturally rise and fall in intensity.

Nature seemed to move at a good, solid pace. The earth wasn't turning faster, the moon and the sun hadn't sped up – it was only the world's system of over-productivity that was going faster and faster, and us along with it. I was beginning to see how the rushing that most of the world was doing – and which I had been a part of – was at a level we are simply not designed for.

Nature trusts the process. And a great reward of surrender is to learn that recovery of any kind is a process. It might be recovery from something big, like a health scare or a divorce, or from something more contained, like a bad day or a hurtful comment. We don't have to constantly try to control our circumstances and berate ourselves for not being better in each moment. We are a process. Loved just by being alive as we are right now.

The world's modern pace was laughably trying to override my nature, leaving no time for this process, or my vulnerability or needs. It was so clear to see, with this ghastly privilege I had of watching the world go by and not being able to partake, that we so often need to stop and check in with ourselves, but like dear rats in a race we keep doing and rushing, chasing our tail, even as things start to pile up. (The number of times I used to say, 'I'll relax when I get this done' – can't just be me?) NO WONDER WE'RE ALL SO KNACKERED! And then when things do pile up, and monsters emerge, we may operate from a fearful place of comparison and self-judgement as everyone else looks okay, and so the masks go back on, pretending we're fine and trying to make ourselves acceptable. We've come to believe that despite being stressed, we can't give in. Bless us. It's a hard pattern to smash, but smash it we must!

Giving In Is Not Giving Up

Ah, giving in. I used to consider this nothing more than giving up. But it's such a lie, MDRC. If we're even remotely facing our monsters, then acceptance and surrender are absolutely not succumbing weakly to a situation. The opposite. In this regard, running away is actually and assuredly giving in. Meeting our worst fears and facing difficult situations are surely infinitely braver than carrying on or numbing away.

I have done some relatively brave things in my life. I have abseiled in the Swiss Alps with Bear Grylls with no head for heights, my violent breaking of wind on national television proving it was not something I found easy – you're welcome. (Although sharing a small tent with Bear and *his* wind after a vegetable curry was almost worse than abseiling . . . as was desperately needing a wee in the middle of the night on a mountain at minus 15 degrees.) I have performed stand-up for 15,000 people at The O2. But, I declare, the bravest thing I have ever had to do was surrender to how I was feeling physically and emotionally when I collapsed for that second time.

Allowing and accepting aren't giving up. Giving up isn't even giving up. Often quitting is right and necessary and braver than anything. It's fine to have gone down the wrong path – who doesn't sometimes?

And so, here I was facing my circumstances so that I could create a better way forward. My sole aim became to come home to my wild, true self, to live free and well. Yes, it's part of my wild self to make things, produce things, go on adventures, make bold moves in love and life. But wildness occurs in rest too. What would a wild beast do if it was wounded? It would hide, go quiet and take time to heal. It would go into 'a cave'.

John, our lovely 'ist', once said that if I could very carefully watch an animal, I would see that *all* they are doing is regulating themselves, getting comfortable and meeting their needs. Always taking the next right action. It was fascinating to watch my dog intently and purely from this point of view. Little Peggy was constantly adjusting her position to get as comfortable as possible. When she was thirsty she drank. When she wanted to go outside she would tell me. After she ate she rested, often taking two or three goes to find the perfect spot, turning and turning into a tighter ball to get as cosy as she dared. Humans don't remotely take such good care of themselves in the quest 'to do'. NO WONDER WE'RE ALL SO KNACKERED!

It boils, yet again, down to the fact that my dog (all animals) doesn't worry about how worthy she is or judge herself based on how well she is doing or being perceived; she just knows she is a beautiful, one-off, glorious creature. It is her solemn duty to look after herself.

I was learning that my true nature, my 'wildness' at this moment in my life was also about stillness, waiting and rest. A state that is natural for us, though the modern world doesn't remind us. And as soon as I did, I realized something that has been a total game-changer for me: getting still is also a dignified adventure.

Who was to say this dark experience wasn't going to be productive? Nature doesn't judge the rain or question the gentle cycle of leaves falling off trees. Nature doesn't grandly think there should be another way. A tree doesn't apologize for its gnarly barren winter branches. It knows it is then that it's doing its greatest work. This could be vital hallowed fallow time.

When You Are Waiting,
You Are Not Doing Nothing

I read a generously honest memoir by Sue Monk Kidd, *When the Heart Waits*, about her mid-life crisis. In it, she wrote, 'We achieve our deepest progress standing still.' But my hand is firmly up again to admit that it took this now ex-productivity junkie a very long time to truly believe that.

I couldn't understand – or trust – that my life would get guidance and direction, or start to unfold, without my forcing it. Without my mind planning and organizing to make change for myself. But here's the remarkable thing, MDRC: I found that when I stopped expending the energy to gird my loins and brace against reality, my body really did start to heal. With nothing else, no magic potions, just the release of not fighting. I was literally breathing better. I got some energy back. Which meant I had room to develop and nurture new ways and qualities of being.

The first deeply important quality that emerged for me was hope. I had the energy to choose hope. It was still something I had to actively choose. Eventually, hope grew, and I got to a place where I knew that, even if I didn't fully heal, I could still have a good life. I could do illness well. I was no longer at war with myself and my situation, and I understood that it was possible to have a peace that transcends all understanding.

The whisperings of the truth were becoming louder. Waiting leads to hope. To my mind, that is one of the most fruitful things you can produce.

To reiterate, this wasn't an easy, laugh-a-minute kind of a time. About the only thing I could do from my bed or chair with any kind of ease was watch films, albeit sometimes with dark glasses because of neurological symptoms from the light sensitivity. But hope meant I was able to start looking for the good. A simple tool I learnt was to do just that: Name the Good. If you're in fear, try looking around where you are. What good can you name? Nice colours in the room? Some beauty out of the window? This simple act can be revolutionary if we are stuck in the negative place of nothing being good enough. Naming the good (usually stroking Peggy's soft fur and having a cup of tea – not at the same time) was the way to keep hope, feel safe, focus on the picnic not the wasps. But that was kind of it. Nothing more marvellous or miraculous (though it felt both). I just decided not to put on a brave face any more. I felt seriously ill, so I would just let myself be so. I felt weak, so I would let myself be so. I felt scared, so I would let myself be so. It wasn't easy. And from it, an ease came.

Acceptance and surrender are the greatest actions you can take when you need to. Surrender is the beginning, not the end. It's the bedrock of transformation and from where all the good stuff comes. It means moments to vitally stop and understand – and perhaps break – the pattern of who we are trying to be, so that we can pick up the pieces of who we actually are. In this case it showed me what I truly believe, that as well as being strong, brave, doing, planning people who can find ways to make a living, get things done and create good work, we are also inherently people of hope, stillness, and trust. We have perhaps forgotten that those are as important as any other trait, if not more.

Waiting really did become an adventure. That's wild to me.

Try Trust

We are nearing the end of Treasure Two, MDRC – and I shall share that the greatest trait I learnt from putting down my armour of fighting against reality and wanting better was ... learning to trust.

I was struck by how little trust I had had in my life. Could I start to really believe there was a force greater than me that I could lean into that would help unfold my life, lead me? That there were people and places that could help me and not let me down? I knew that would be the biggest game-changer if I could, that it was a lack of trust which meant I kept carrying my own burdens. Or trying to hold it together. Think about the language of 'holding it all together' or 'soldiering on'. Exhausting.

So, I chose to trust. I handed over my trial to what I understand to be God, and trusted I was loved and looked after. That the answers would come. That the next right steps would be clear and possible. That I would have the courage to follow them. Trust is different for all of us. Some people focus on the beauty of nature to make them feel held and safe, or a pet, or a person who has recently passed away – someone or something to feel like an anchor that has their good will in their heart. Others find trusting another human much harder; their experience has led them to believe that people aren't to be trusted. Which is why I say 'Try trust'. It was easier for me to start with God. For others it will be the opposite. I certainly always found nature a surefire route into more calm and trust.

MDRC, do you notice that your worries are where your problems are? That might sound silly or facetious. But think about it for a moment. Are there areas in your life that just tick along all right, that always work out or near enough? Now think about all the things that you are fearful won't work out – aren't you instantly more negative and stressed? And that's when things are likely to go wrong. Because there's no trust.

In the past I'd always trusted that somehow, despite the odds being firmly against it, it was possible I could become a comedy actress. That didn't mean there wasn't hard work, sacrifice and difficulty in trying it, but it did mean that I just let it unfold without expectation, and therefore considerably less stress. I handed it over – if it happened, it happened. I was similar about trusting I may find my person and fall in love. As far back as I can remember, I had this niggling sense of, *I think I will marry at fifty-one and that will do me well.* Even when that felt like far too far away, I didn't give it much more thought. If someone came along earlier, or didn't at all, then fine either way. There's not much I can control there either. I was therefore never particularly angry or sad that I hadn't found that solid relationship. Even though I wanted it.

However, as I got older, and that want turned into a deep longing, meeting someone seemed less and less realistic (especially when bringing an illness to the party). My trust began to fade. It was no coincidence that as my trust faded, I felt less hope and more aloneness.

The thing I never trusted was my health. It was therefore the area of my life I was most stressed by. I needed to keep choosing hope and trust, day by day. Another exciting heavy revvy came to me: if trust comes from surrender, and if the opposite of surrender is ignoring what our body needs, ignoring our emotional needs, forcing ourselves to be stronger than we are, continuing to help others rather than saying when we need help, then trust includes the need to trust ourselves. We cannot trust ourselves to take care of ourselves if we are not taking care of ourselves! I was determined my new-found trust would develop a faithfulness. That is, a loyalty to myself with whatever I might be experiencing. We have to belong to ourselves too, I suppose.

Faithfulness became my watchword for this treasure. Our carry on fixing culture is the opposite of faithfulness. And what is there to fix about us, MDRC, thank you, please? We are exquisite. We might just need a fallow time for some maintenance, give ourselves a good service (sounds wrong . . . moving on . . .).

Be your own loyal faithful friend. Life surely feels a lot kinder.

I now have a healthy dollop of faithfulness to hope and trust in myself and life which I would never have thought possible, and it wouldn't have happened without 'giving in'.

Finally, A Moment of Surrender

After that second collapse, I was the most ill I have been. Yet one day I took some breaths, named some good around me, noticed how comfortable my bed was, how kindly soft the duvet was on top of me, and remembered that day in May when I had felt the sun on me, and the voice saying I could give up the fight, and I relaxed into my bed. I just let it all kind of be. I didn't force myself to do it, it just finally came.

I remember saying to myself, out loud because it felt significant, 'Wow, Miranda, that was finally a true moment of surrender.' Sure, I wanted answers, and sure, I wanted it to be over. I was frustrated by my small, incapacitated life. I really missed my friends and my work. But whenever I saw what those thoughts were doing to me – as my muscles tensed and the bracing meant I couldn't find the good and joy in the moment, all clearly making me more tired – I slowly changed tack. I trusted that this part of my life, however confusing right now, would unfold. I accepted that I was not able to get in a car and go and see the bluebells. But the bluebells would be there next year and the year after that.

I didn't have to accept my suffering as such, but I could accept how it was making me feel, where it was leading me, and what I needed in the moment to thrive the best I could. Sure, I would always have goals and dreams, but if they happened, they happened. And now, at the top of my list is a trust in whatever life throws at me. I have to practise every day, but I'm surrendered.

Lying there in bed that day, I took away the dramatic, fearful story of being ill. I kindly turned to myself and, as I would to a young child going through something, said, 'Hello, I'm sorry you're going through this. How can I help? What's our next right step?'

P.S. 'We Can't All Just Stop To Drink Tea And Watch Films'

MDRC, I would hate you to think that surrender means we need the privilege that is a cosy house, a perfect loving relationship, finances, an understanding boss and all those luxuries we feel we may need to surrender, stop and rest. Not everyone has those ingredients. I certainly didn't have many of them.

I'm also aware that surrender may sound like I mean lying about on a plush sofa, with all the scatter cushions and fleecy blankets a person may desire, watching TV all day. It isn't. It's an active stance; a turning towards a new frame of mind. Sometimes it might lead to total bed rest where necessary. Sometimes it might lead to delegating aspects of our life if we can. But if circumstances mean people have or want to keep going in their roles in life, surrender can absolutely happen within that. And that's often the best way. A structure is incredibly helpful (I certainly found I floundered losing one), and families and jobs give good focus beyond difficulty. You don't need luxury to surrender. We are scared and alone, and need to create moments of stillness to try acceptance and trust. We need a friend. In ourselves. And hopefully another too.

Treasure Three

Feel, Grieve, Let the Past Be the Past

TREASURES PICKED UP: Allowing expression, grieving to move your story on, taking up your space, listening to the messages of feelings, finding safety to feel

PATTERNS SMASHED: Toxic positivity, repression, hardening to present how you think you 'should', avoiding anger

WATCHWORD: Peace

SOUNDTRACK: 'Flashdance . . . What a Feeling' by Irene Cara

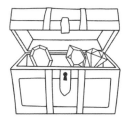

Feel, Grieve, Let the Past Be the Past

Goodbye, Peggy

When my beloved-beyond-all-compare dog Peggy died, I found myself in a state of grief I had never felt before. I was emoting, sharing, expressing, sobbing – and freely so. The death of a pet, I realized, is understood and accepted. That said, it was a bit of a shock to find the loss of my dog in the broadsheet headlines! I could have been embarrassed, but I took it as testimony to the immense power of our canine friends.

Peggy taught me many lessons throughout her life – dogs do, if you let them. It's part of their job, alongside providing us with unconditional love and loyalty (and, of course, developing the skill to pick up poo in one deft manoeuvre). And they do so with a grounded simplicity. Without a whirring human brain, they are able to be present for the one thing on their doggy to-do list – follow their human around and show them they love them At All Times. With a human companion you can share experiences, but you can't know if they're also thinking about what chore they have to do next or mulling on something they are worried about. A dog is wholly present with no such concerns. I suppose there could be a deeply vain Bichon Frisé worrying about the bow in her hair not looking quite right, but I doubt it . . .

On any occasion I was sick or injured, dear little fluffy Peggy would lie on my lap or, more often than not, right next to the place that hurt. I was instantly calmer, breathed easier and slower, the lack of resistance to what was happening relaxing my body so that it could heal. To this end, Peggy was perhaps my first teacher in surrender and acceptance.

It was during the first days, when the grief was pounding to a surprising degree, that I realized the pain was about losing that loving presence in its purest form. My grief was amplified by remorse over not being as present with her as I could have been – and absolutely wanted to have been – in her last few months. I had become consumed with the illnesses I was facing. I had let illness become my identity. Disaster.

The first morning after she died, I would have done anything to have her back – to experience the classic enthusiastic Peggy morning greeting (even though, before I had fully woken up, it might involve a paw plant straight on my nose). So often of late I would give her a cursory stroke and smile; I'd never ignore her – she was too wonderful to ignore – but I'd take her for granted.

The regret of wishing I had spent more time just stroking her, just lying next to her, was a huge wake-up call to acknowledge that I had been instead worrying about how sick I was and therefore getting sicker. As I mourned all the joyful times we had had together, just me and Peggy, I realized, too, that in the last few years those adventures had become less and less frequent. I was grieving the car journeys and how I loved her sitting on the passenger seat asleep or looking up at me as I sang my heart out! Finding a grassy verge at the service station to pee on – her, not me. All the routines. So many of which we hadn't done for so long because my dear body was unable to. We had rarely been apart. I missed her lying beside me as I wrote. I grieved the routine of sitting down after breakfast at my laptop, with a clear purpose for the day ahead, and then a couple of hours later us both stirring as we knew it was walk time. Walkies were as much of an excitement for me as they were for her. With a dog you are somehow spiritually connected to your animal's joy for their surrounds. Your heart soars as they look around to check you are still with them. Always tethered, never too far apart. My last proper countryside walk with Peggy was years before she died.

Peggy's death forced me to face all that I was mourning from illness. The waking up to *that*, however painful, was also a start to healing. Perhaps she left to get my attention. Perhaps grief of any kind is so confounding that it wakes us up to what else we may not have noticed we were needing or missing.

It certainly drew attention to the fact that grieving the loss of a pet was the first time I had freely emoted – and been listened to – in a while. Which in turn drew attention to the fact that I hadn't grieved my full diagnosis, the one I had been searching for and had finally received a few months before Peggy's death. Post-diagnosis, I had sniffled through a couple of days before unconsciously going back into a 'keep calm and carry on' mode.

Why was I allowing myself Peggy grief but clamming up about my diagnosis? If I thought about trying to put a lid on Peggy's death, I immediately felt that familiar bracing tightness around my muscles. It's bad enough, isn't it, when you need to do a little cry but stop yourself and that tight lump in your throat comes on.

Being able to share and express my grief over Peggy made it more bearable. My heart healed, and relatively quickly. But why hadn't I done the same with my diagnosis, with all the disappointments of illness? I found the answer in this treasure. We're still in pretty murky territory, MDRC, but, as promised, the treasures shall get more playful and peaceful ... In fact, 'peace' became my watchword for this, our third treasure together.

I learnt that the Hebrew word for peace – 'shalom' – is not a simple state of absence of problems. Instead, it means a totality or completeness, fulfilment, wholeness, harmony, security and well-being. Yes, please, thank you, please, wouldn't mind me some of *that*. Unfortunately, it turns out, that meant learning how to grieve and feel – help! But, if the gift of dogs are their wholehearted faithful loving presence, this was what I wanted Peggy's death to teach me: how to be present with my feelings so that I could be vulnerable and present with others, too.

The only way to get to that was to go through the darkness.

Diagnosis

Slowly, the grief of all that I had missed with Peggy due to my illness became greater than the loss of my beloved dog. Initially I felt a little guilty about that – surely, I should grieve the loss of another creature more than my own disappointments? And that pointed to part of the problem: what we feel we have the right to emote, grieve and share, and what we don't.

I received a clear diagnosis for my three-plus-decades-long mystery of challenging health a few months after the first Covid lockdown. I had Zoom calls with two experts who both confirmed – from a delightful smorgasbord of blood tests – that I had been living with a constant, reactivated Lyme disease. It transpired that Lyme – a bacterial infection – would have most likely come from an infected tick when I was just fourteen. I had picked up – what seemed like then – a nasty flu-like bug while living in Virginia, USA (my father was working in Washington, DC). Virginia is a well-known Lyme disease hotspot – but it wasn't known or treated as it is now. And here's what I didn't know: most people can get an acute disease/virus/infection, and their immune system dispels it over a few weeks of being very unwell (like Covid, for most). Or they take specific antibiotics to treat it. For others, like me, the immune system is never able to fully detoxify it. This can be due – as it was in my case – to a gene that increases susceptibility to immune dysfunction and the fact that the disease was never identified at the time. The body goes back to *just* enough health so that you think you are recovered, but the virus actually remains active. From then on, the immune system doesn't have capacity to cope with other bugs that one naturally gets over the course of a life, meaning that more viruses stay active in one's body instead of passing through – some they found in me included Epstein-Barr/glandular fever/herpes/shingles and some other nasties I don't care to remember for they all sounded so awful. I switched off altogether when the doctors said, 'They tend to attack the brain.' Urgh, please . . . But that's what happens if treatment is delayed with Lyme – you can end up with neurological issues, nerve damage and trouble with memory and concentration.

As an aside, I have always said diseases should be given jollier names! For example, let's call gonorrhoea 'Burning Love' or jaundice 'Sunshine Yellow'. Though, a lot of lovely plants sound like diseases. I was very alarmed when someone asked me to look at their blooming ceanothus – I didn't know what I was about to be privy to . . . I'm avoiding . . . Back to my endless diagnoses . . .

I ended up with, as the doctor described it, thick blood, heavy with toxins. (A very ME (Myalgic encephalomyelitis) kind of picture.) This made it feel as though I had flu every day (to put it mildly). When energy cells become severely depleted, the immune system further dysregulates, unable to rid itself of simple daily toxins. Each year it gets harder, as more complicated secondary conditions emerge from the inflammation – such as autoimmune and gut problems, heavy metal toxicity, histamine issues (the rashes were also delightful – medically known as urticaria, but I called them my 'Jolly Dot-to-Dot Body Art' and PoTS, or Postural tachycardia syndrome – if you know you know and hello to you if you do – there's hope. The latter I just childishly call 'Pots and Pans'). For me, however, it was the unnerving neurological symptoms that I had got initially, aged fourteen, from Lyme, which I always found particularly hard to deal with. And they got considerably worse as I headed into my forties. As did the fatigue from the cell depletion. Yup, all delightful.

I got off that Zoom call, pulled my laptop shut and sat there, still and aghast. So many emotions. I was shocked, but I also immediately felt a deep well of sadness and disappointment – for over three decades I'd *KNOWN* there was something wrong. I recalled all the times I'd told different doctors, 'I feel toxic and poisoned,' or, 'It's like I have flu every day but I don't have a temperature.' (It's amazing how the body can sometimes literally tell us what's going on.) I felt anger rising at the times I'd been told I must have agoraphobia. I would try and treat it as such, when, as it turned out, it was the lack of energy and the extreme light and sound sensitivity that made my body crash when going out to be in any kind of activity or stimulating environment.

Even with a diagnosis, it felt hard to know how to share the news. I still had a chronic, not acute, illness. I was still, to an outsider, 'just tired all the time'. TATT. I was debilitated but also lucky in so many ways – I feared being perceived as complaining. I realize now why so many experts and therapists became so after their own recoveries – I think in particular of the help I got from the Optimum Health Clinic, and why they, among others, call it 'chronic *invisible* illness'. The invisibility is part of the problem. After long Covid this is more understood; I can say I have long Lyme and people understand a little more easily. Year on year, the 'chronic fatigue, ME, long post-viral condition' bracket is getting more visible. I hope so, for it is a very real, severe, physical illness.

I stared at my laptop for a while and eventually walked very slowly to a garden shed at my parents' house, which was where I had spent 'the Covid years' (not in their shed, they allowed me in the house!). I sat down on a chair and cried a little. But in the main, I was so overwhelmed by the size of this news – the way my life story suddenly needed to be rewritten – that I remained open-mouthed and quiet. All the years of knowing there was something wrong and being silenced, all the years I would apologize or push on because I had been told it was a weirdly manifesting anxiety attack, all the years my illness could have been prevented (90 per cent of those suffering from Lyme disease can recover fully), the missed opportunities, the losses, the aloneness, the fear of wondering 'What next?' It was too much to settle on one feeling. I let myself sniffle for a couple of days and then I 'pulled myself together'.

Do I Have the Right To Grieve?

I can see now that I didn't feel I had permission to grieve my diagnosis, in part due to the acute awareness of my privileges – I had to remind myself that there is no way to measure what makes one person's pain worse or better than another's. As grief expert David Kessler says, 'What each person is going through is the worst thing that they have been through.' We all have the right to grieve.

A question was forming. What if we get stuck in some illnesses and situations because we don't have the ways to, or don't allow ourselves to, grieve and feel them? We aren't letting them move through us. Umm . . .

All Hail The 'Ists'

Sure enough, all the 'ists' on this matter told me that if we don't honour and release our pain, wounds, upsets, disappointments, we will only relive them. It's so ingrained in us (well, I speak for myself) to ignore and push away what we perceive to be the difficult emotions. We force the positives instead. But tactics to avoid discomfort don't work. That energy of feeling (emotion is energy in motion) might be suppressed, but it's still fizzing away, unreleased, in the body. I suppose I always thought that if I wasn't feeling an emotion, then it wasn't there, so it couldn't have an effect. Oh, how wrong I could be! Emotion sits there, within our cells, our organs, our nervous, immune and hormonal systems, adding stress within the body. This can then cause inflammation (which, when ongoing, is definitely NOT the friend of a healthy body).

As trauma expert Bessel van der Kolk astutely said, *The Body Keeps the Score*. Is it any wonder so many people have tiredness, tight shoulders, jaw pain, headaches, lower back pain and migraines? It's not just the lack of an ergonomic chair and computer set-up, it's also because many of us are gripping on to maintain a good façade. On the masks go so as not to risk being judged or unloved for having feelings the world has deemed as less acceptable.

For years I was averse to having to feel anything but happy and positive. It turns out, MDRC, that this is not humanly or scientifically possible. Apparently – and sorry to hit you with this because I didn't like hearing it at first – if we suppress one end of our emotional spectrum, we can't but suppress the whole. We end up in a bland middle ground.

If there is physical pain, chronic issues, disturbed sleep, digestive problems, discontent, there is likely a dear little feeling rumbling around that needs to come out. If only we could just fart out an emotion. Ironically, that's one thing I do freely release. I didn't want to pick up the phone and howl angrily about my diagnoses to a friend, though I had every right, and I sometimes even stifle irritability, but I will happily do a massive fart in public. (That's public-school education in England for you – repress emotions but it's fine to talk about poo!)

So, there we have it. It really is better out than in. All the 'ists' say that what comes out of you doesn't make you sick, it's what stays in there that does. I was starting to confront the possibility that part of my ongoing diagnoses might relate to some emotional repression.

'Don't Get Emotional, We're Not Spanish!'

That was a line from the upper-class mother character in the first episode of my sitcom. It was quite an obvious way to help the audience understand her character, but the way Patricia Hodge said it made it very funny. It's perhaps something only a British audience can really understand – there truly are some who go queasy at the thought of having an emotion! There are many who were brought up to keep quiet and be polite at all costs. That being raucous in any way is unseemly.

So, for anyone thinking this silly line was a jibe at the Spanish, not remotely. I'm quite sure that the healthy Mediterranean lifestyle is not just the diet of olive oil and tomatoes but also that emotions are released from the body. I'm sure that's why Italians might be able to eat pasta and pizza and have fewer heart attacks. They can have an argument, emote their opinions, gesticulate irritations, and laugh and hug the next minute. They let it out. That, to me, seems natural and truthful. There's an honest wildness about it that you don't always see in Britain. (I suspect all the olive oil in Spain couldn't smooth the arteries of rage repression.) I should add, the line wasn't a jibe against any uptightness in us Brits either. There is much to applaud about our stoicism, duty, keep-calm-and-carry-on-ness. Often these are necessary and noble traits. Just not all the time.

But we can't just suddenly say to someone with culturally ingrained, buttoned-up emotions, 'Come on, just let it all out.' As I delved into the 'ists' on this treasure, I saw it would take some learning and unlearning. Many a pattern to smash. Ready to dive in with me, MDRC? Start feeling some feelings? Don't panic, I had to go super gently. So much so I simply started with what a feeling is. If you're worried, then perhaps sing 'Jerusalem' or the national anthem and grab a Victoria sponge. Soon it will all be a piece of cake . . . (thank you).

What Is A Feeling?

Feelings are conscious reactions to emotions. Stick with me, MDRC, I found this so super helpful to learn. Emotions are subconscious energy – raw, immediate responses to the moment. (I mean, I did not know that – what a revelation.) Let me explain with an example. If someone hides behind a door and jumps out at you, you will likely scream without even thinking about it. Getting a fright, you might leap out of the way, put your hand over your mouth, feel a bit shaky, perhaps hot and flushed in your shock, as you recoil from what your brain cleverly automatically thinks is a threat. All that energy in motion comes from the primal part of the brain that protects us. That's emotion. Pure physical energy that gets expressed in a number of ways, biologically, facially, with noise and language.

Now, keep concentrating on my lesson, MDRC, as it gets more interesting and helpful (*It's not possible, Miranda*, I hear you say . . .) – feelings are influenced by these emotions but they come from our mental, conscious thoughts. Feelings are the meaning we put to the emotion. Don't you think that's fascinating? I wondered why I didn't know it before. So, feelings might end up being stories we've created based on past events or fears of the future. For example, if my friend jumps out at me and I scream and get a fright, then I could feel joyful, playful, excited because I love surprises, and it makes me feel loved to have that kind of playful relationship. The initial shock and scream then goes into warm feelings of laughter and connection. However, for another, or on another day, getting a shock like that, with all the energy that emotion creates, might lead to feelings of fear, upset, stress. It might remind me of something in the past, knowingly or unknowingly, and it might be misinterpreted as a mean action by my friend, not a silly, loving one. Those are the feelings created from emotion. All happening within a blink of an eye.

114

I wondered why any of us had become so afraid of or removed from this part of our humanness. So vital to know. So natural.

Emotions are the primal, instinctive, subconscious bodily responses to the here and now. Feelings are our mental thoughts about an emotion, and not necessarily the truth of the situation. Ah, okay, I thought, so that's why people can get stuck. If our minds are always in stories from our past, our phobias, our beliefs of inadequacy, or whatever it is – like assuming a friend was being mean instead of loving with a prank – then emotions get misconstrued, and we become scared of our feelings and numb out.

But we are emotional beings, and without our emotions, we couldn't survive. We need the energy of fear, for example, to help us leap out of the way of a fast-moving vehicle. It's always reassuring to remember that there are only seven key human emotions, all of which are designed to keep us alive: joy, anger, fear, sadness, contempt, disgust and surprise. We are feeling beings, otherwise we would have no meaning. We are feeling beings with meanings (just felt like a little rhyme). We can't not feel. It's impossible. We might as well discover them, get used to them, learn how to deal with them then, mightn't we? Even enjoy them.

They are part of who we are. They make life richer and more beautiful. They are honest. It all spoke to that deep longing of mine not to have a bland world full of polite bland people avoiding what they were taught were negative emotions and putting on a polite bland sheen of polite blandness to be loved. I want everyone to be able to be their wild selves. I was galvanized to keep digging.

First, I'm off for a dance break. Joyously, and I jest ye not, research has proved how good dancing is for releasing stuck emotions and stress – I know! Naturally, I'm putting on 'Flashdance . . . What a Feeling'. I just looked up the lyrics. They tell you to move from fear and steel to allowing your feelings. Because of course you make it happen with your passion so you can dance right through life. Speaking song lyrics is always a bit funny.

Childhood

Welcome back, MDRC, I'm quite sweaty. That was quite the routine. I often think I should charge for admission to my dance antics at home. There would be a rush on tickets such is the gay abandon of my performance style and the rogue and revolutionary use of props. I just did quite the manoeuvre with a laundry basket. Moving on . . .

It's a deeper dive into the emotional field. But I found it utterly vital to know, again wondering why on earth I didn't before. (By the way, if you are in a particularly difficult time in your life and want to move to a jollier treasure, feel free to skip along to Treasure Seven or Eight, for example. You might have a couple of spoilers, but go to whichever treasure feels good in the moment.)

Here goes with our deeper dive. We can't ignore that we have each been, at one time in our life, a child. (Don't say you don't learn from me.) We all, regardless of our current status here on earth, even if we are now a leading world public figure, were once a tiny little fragile naked baby. Forgive me,

116

MDRC, if you are now imagining Putin in nappies. Forgive me, too, if you weren't imagining Putin in nappies, but you now are, which is the more likely scenario.

We all started out as vulnerable, fragile, tiny beings with the potential to develop into the loving, uniquely made beings that we are, and how we were raised, what our first few months and few years were witness to, will have had a profound effect on our future.

This was probably one of the most eye-opening and important revelations I gained in this metaphorical cave I was wading through. A real treasure from 'ists' like Gabor Maté, Peter Levine, Stephen Porges, Susan David, Pat Ogden, Pete Walker (and so many others). To survive we need a loving attachment to a caregiver to feed us, clothe us, give us shelter, physical touch, show us love and gently guide our early development. As our brains develop, we need that care figure to make us feel safe, so that the survival part of our brain that produces fear for emergencies doesn't get stuck in that mode. To develop a healthy nervous system we need to be loved and approved of in all aspects of our development in order to create that felt sense of safety. We need to feel safe enough to put boundaries up, to learn to say no, express ourselves. The trouble is, not everyone has that security – I read a statistic that suggested half of the world's population has problems stemming from a lack of safety in early development. There might be some very simple ways that our brains detected danger: from being left to cry for too long, from a mother with a stressful pregnancy so cortisol levels start high from the off (cortisol being the steroid hormone that helps the body regulate stress), from hearing shouting and arguing. Whatever it is, for us to survive, we have to adapt, and quick. This is amazing information, MDRC – we are programmed to placate our caregivers to find a way to attach to them safely. If that is to be quiet and to not share how we feel as we noticed it was only then we get attention, we shut up and possibly shut down. If that is through showing our parents what we have achieved because that's the only time they praise us, we might develop a pattern of perfectionism. If that is being as helpful as we can, even if we are totally ignoring our own needs, we might develop people-pleasing habits.

It was a fascinating, lightning-bolt kind of a moment for me that we are all dear children who had to adapt to feel safe and loved, and that sometimes that adaptation isn't healthy and remains programmed into us for our adult lives.

And bless us, because being a child is terrifying at the best of times. Every day we face something new. We might be innocently taken to the park aged two or three when walking still isn't the most natural thing in the world, and for the first time be confronted by a swan! Imagine coming across a gargantuan white-winged creature with loud, flappy, flippery feet and a hissy orange beak. No wonder we need looking after. No wonder we need lots of rest. No wonder we need physical protection, to be held, looked at with smiles. We need constant reassurance these things are safe. And we need that now too. We might be grown up, we might be adults with responsibilities, but there are still some things we will feel scared about. We have always had needs, and we always will, and it's terrifying to us when they aren't met (many of us likely don't even know what our needs are, let alone how to meet them and look after ourselves).

To conclude the heavy revvy (heavy revelation) of this treasure: if we hide our feelings to fit in and be loved as a little child, that's initially a very clever way to find security, but ultimately, if we take that into adulthood, then we remain living in a subconscious pattern of fear. Our brains store our early attachment stories; there's nothing wrong with you for being wired anxiously or living in patterns you don't want to be in – it's literally not your fault. In fact, the opposite: you were an amazing child who learnt how to survive. Blooming well done you, MDRC. Plus, the 'ists' reassured me that we can dismantle the old unhelpful patterns. Yay and phew!

The Girl Who Was Scared Of the Dog

However excited I was by all this learning – because I felt sure it would relate to my physical health issues – I had to take regular breaks (sometimes days or more) and that would mean a chance to reflect upon times with my darling Peggy. I remembered once sitting on a bridge over a small stream when a couple with two young children approached. Dear Peggles rushed up to them with a small bark and made a bee-line for the older child, clearly wanting a cuddle. Though the younger child rushed forward to play with Peggy, the older child held her mother's hand, recoiling as Peggy leapt up at her face. I was about to go over to the sweet girl, bend down and explain that Peggy loved her and would never hurt her, but I appreciated that it might feel scary. Then her mother suddenly stridently said, 'You can't *possibly* be scared of this little fluffball, I mean honestly!' I don't think she was annoyed with her child, perhaps embarrassed by her at worst. But those words pierced me, as much as they clearly did the girl. She shrank in stature, turned away and clearly wanted to cry.

There it was. The simple way an innocent, well-meaning invalidation of a child's feeling of fear can lead to further fear. I didn't realize that day sitting on the bridge that I was getting a great therapeutic example that a child (though it can happen at any time in life) may not feel safe to express fear the next time she feels it, because she was made to feel stupid for feeling it with a dog. We are often more scared to feel the feeling than have the feeling itself.

Little girl, I wonder where you are now. Please know you were absolutely in your right to be afraid of Peggy. If a dog my height jumped up in my face and I hadn't been told it wouldn't bite my nose off, I would probably scream and never go outside again. I think you were more sensible and more brave than your younger sister just running towards a strange ball of fluff. Little girl, there was nothing wrong with you.

'What's Not To Be Happy About?'

That little girl being forced to be happy about Peggy's meaty breath in her face was also a therapeutic example of the next thing I learnt from the 'ists', called 'toxic positivity'. Another lesson incoming, MDRC. (*I can't wait Miranda*, I hear you say . . .) If our so-called negative emotions are not allowed or

120

if they become scary to us, we naturally try to maintain some kind of cheer.

The culture I grew up in meant that if I was having a moment of feeling stressed or frustrated and shared a little snippet of that, the response was usually 'chin up', 'keep going', 'look at all you have to be happy about' or 'you're okay, it'll be fine'.

However well-meaning (and I'm sure I've said similar myself), I see now that those responses force a sheen of positivity over something that likely needed to be felt and heard and expressed and moved through (which might happen very quickly and easily – I'm not suggesting we constantly over-share, or grind to a halt in endless lamenting and wailing). 'Go and grab the day', 'be positive', 'be polite', 'be brave', 'take on the world' – all of these can be good things. But when they stop us from having a full emotional experience without shame, when we worry more about letting the mood down, or not being liked, or being a burden, then we're creating a toxic positive culture in which suppression becomes the only option.

How flipping exhausting is it to always have to be 'on form'? That feels like a cage to me. What does it even mean anyway? Surely 'on form' is just how we are and who we are, and that will vary every day in so much as what we experience will affect how we react to things. Some days I might be quieter and more reflective and that's okay.

I am certainly always going to be a sensitive person. I feel things very intensely, from galloping with excitement and when I feel surges of hope, to my heart hurting if I hear an argument or someone being told off! I startle easily and have a vivid imagination, which means if I am swimming in the sea and something brushes my skin, I will scream and assume it's a deadly snake even if it's in England, where there are no deadly snakes. It's always a stick or a plastic bag or at worst a piece of seaweed! I will cry with joy at the beauty of a puppy bounding or a sunset. If someone I love feels encouraged and like they have achieved something great, then my heart swells. And I cry. And then jump up and down. And then wee. When someone surprises me, I'm nervited – nervous and excited (you have to know me very well to get away with a surprise that could work).

Was I told I'm just too sensitive? YES.

Am I too sensitive? NO, no, no and all the nos in the Kingdom of No.

It's who I am. It's how I'm made. I can't change it. I don't choose to get weepy at a limping swan in front of someone who has just recognized me off of the telly. I'd rather not! To that end, in the light of my diagnosis, I understood quite how tiring it would be on those already struggling energy cells to suppress my sensitivity. (The sensitivity I now love and celebrate.) And I had a little weep, knowing I often had.

Stuck In The Mud

A few years after my diagnosis – spoiler alert, but I hope it serves as encouragement for anything you might be going

122

through – I grew stronger (the treasures did work). And one day I had the energy for a trip to the seaside. I can't tell you how beautiful the sea looks after years stuck inside. A friend and I rented a kayak and a tiny RIB boat with an engine (when we wanted a paddling break) for a nice potter up a beautiful creek. It was relaxing for a short while until the engine on the little boat, at this point also towing the kayak, cut out. The tide was going out rapidly and we knew that getting back to our jetty against the tide and wind, and with the deep, sinking mud of the estuary slowly revealing itself, was going to be a bit of a feat. We tried to use the kayak paddle for the boat but we weren't making any headway – by which I mean we were staying still, by which I mean we were going backwards despite trying to put our muscles into going forward. We were up shit creek with the wrong sort of paddles (not sorry for that). It was time for me to transfer to the kayak and try and tow us in (it was a single-person kayak unfortunately). What I thought would be a relatively simple segue from a RIB boat to a kayak WAS NOT. I did not make a steady manoeuvre and plopped (good word, PLOP) into the water (screaming at the 'snakes'!). It was only thigh-high, if that, but now I was screaming because if you try and stand up in very deep mud, especially when you weigh quite a lot, you start sinking and naturally topple over. You then, it turns out, lose your Crocs. My friend was in hysterics – but I most assuredly was not! I couldn't get securely on to the kayak as we were being pulled gently back down the creek. I kept saying to my friend, deeply seriously (which made her laugh even more), 'Stop laughing, it's not funny until I'm in!' I was happy to find the funny side of this adventure, but I was feeling a little scared and very out of breath (this was quite the escapade for someone having recently been bedbound and still getting the odd attack of PoTS!), and I wanted some kind of safety before I did.

I share this little story because it was my way of clearly understanding that we adult humans need to feel safe, as much as our dear childhood selves. It's only when we feel safe – that is, when our primal limbic brain is not on high alert – that we can freely connect to others, feel emotions, feel loved, create, challenge ourselves (though, ideally for me, not getting stuck in tidal mud). That is often why we don't express emotion. Because we don't feel in a safe enough environment. We need the right people, and a sense of belonging and esteem in ourselves, to feel and express whatever we feel.

I needed to get safely into the kayak before I could laugh with my friend (which I did, as well as putting stripes of mud on my cheeks to feel like an Amazonian warrior princess – obviously).

The Date

One time in a human's life when we definitely need to feel safe to be vulnerable enough to share, cry, grieve or even laugh loudly is when we start a new friendship or romantic relationship. The latter in particular means that we likely want to portray a wholly presentable version of ourselves and hold back on the full truth for a while! (Though I stand by dropping our masks as soon as we dare . . .)

Now, here's a big twist of my tale, MDRC. I got the chance to experience this vulnerability as regards a possibly romantic relationship. Because – wait for it – I went on a date. I KNOW! For the first time in ... Doesn't matter, moving on ... Truly a twist because one minute I'm grieving my diagnosis in a shed during a pandemic and the next I'm telling you that I met a boy, worthy to consider an 'appointment' with! I KNOW. Let's just get a little bit of perspective though. I wasn't suddenly sipping cocktails at a hotel bar in a sexy trouser suit or anything. This was a year or so on from 'the shed' but little had changed globally, pandemic-wise, or personally, housebound health-wise (we are very much pre being up shit creek!). The date therefore consisted of a cup of tea in my sitting room, with some social distancing in force, passing biscuits to each other at arm's length. In many ways, it made it feel more relaxed. There's no fear of how to partake of the often ghastly first-kiss lunge when we have to be two metres apart! However, having met The Boy once briefly, and having chatted to him a couple of times on the phone (very nineties of us), I was already pretty taken by him. I therefore decided I was going to practise not hiding myself or any natural emotions. I was going to be vulnerable to forge as honest a connection as I could. As I opened the door to him, my heart was racing for three reasons: One, I WAS ON SOME KIND OF DATE FOR THE FIRST TIME IN ... Doesn't matter, moving on ... Two, he was very lovely to look at – can we take a moment to breathe in the dashingness of the salt-and-pepper greying hair look on a fine-featured man? Three, I was going to be open and honest in this new way. He knew that my health wasn't good, that I didn't have energy to go on a walk or anything, and so ensconcing myself firmly on and in the sofa wasn't too vulnerable. But the first thing that felt a little awkward was allowing him to make the second cup of tea. Despite not having the energy, there was still that instinct to override and leap up because 'I should host'. Thoughts came in like, *I look weak*, or, *I look like a diva*. But I stayed firmly put. Go me!

And, MDRC, please note *second* cup of tea. Yes, we'd been chatting and getting on very well and easily, thank you very much, please. I didn't police myself from getting a little teary about Peggy when he asked, and it led to a beautiful, natural, connecting moment when he told me about a dog he'd lost ten years earlier, and how sad he still feels when he thinks of that goodbye. He too welled up a little. (I do like a man who weeps with ease!) The second cup of tea segued into a take-away pizza. And it was via said pizza that things nearly came a cropper.

We brought the pizzas from the delivery man into the kitchen and opened the boxes. My pizza had done that thing of shunting itself towards one end of the box, ending up in a crumpled mess. I found myself saying, properly grumpy and like a petulant teenager, 'Oh, that's SO annoying, all my toppings are all over the place, I'm really pissed off.' He looked at me, for I didn't immediately 'dishonestly' laugh it off – I genuinely was annoyed by my shunted pizza! MDRC, this was my chance. My chance not to apologize, just be an idiot who was unnecessarily cross about her wonky pizza. I went on, 'It's just I was SOOOO looking forward to my pizza, they are such a treat, I love them SOOOO MUCH' – it's true but I had never been so publicly exuberant about it! 'Oh, look' – yes, I carried on – 'all that mozzarella curled up against the cardboard, it actually looks so sad. I don't think' – oh yes, MDRC, I was *still* carrying on – 'I will enjoy it as much now. It's like a pizza trying to be a calzone or vice versa, look at the poor thing.' A pause. Either he'd think I was childish and over the top and weird, or he wouldn't (to be fair, when life becomes very small the excitement of a pizza becomes HUGE). He replied, 'Oh, I totally get it, I was worryingly excited about a pizza delivery.' (I do like people who get excited about food.) And he continued, 'Also, I wasn't going to say, but I'm a little pissed off that mine isn't that hot.'

It may be such a silly example to you, MDRC, especially if you are from any culture that just simply expresses (hello to you my Spanish friends), but being grumpy for a silly reason on a first date was completely new. And it FELT GREAT. So freeing. No masks! (Which were entirely dropped when I myself dropped a bit of tomato on my chest. I laughed, 'Oops, landed on my, what I call, breast shelf.')

I knew that our weep over our dogs, our grump and then giggles about the pizza, the silent joy in which we then ate it, were all making for the best connection this first date could, whether we would see each other again or not. Yup, it truly FELT GREAT.

Feeling Good

Sometimes, it might feel like you are battling upstream, against the tide, as you navigate feelings that you have suppressed for years, as you understand why you have suppressed them, not to mention the how and why you need to release them. But generally, all I can say is that I thought it would be way harder than it ended up being. I saw that by allowing a fuller range of emotion, I was feeling more joy and hope and other good stuff that may also have been quashed with repression.

Although this isn't a 'how-to' book (I hope to do an accompanying workbook), I wanted to share here a few things I found helpful, in case you're in a dark patch of life, MDRC.

The first thing is to keep remembering that you are a human (again, don't say you don't learn from me) and humans have nervous systems that need to feel safe. You might surmise that I felt instinctively trusting of The Boy. (I wouldn't necessarily stomp into a work meeting and rage to my colleagues about a disappointing pizza or indeed quite how angry the buffering wheel of doom on my computer makes me – it just happened – still can't surrender to *that*.) But I had to learn to create that safety for myself too. If I kept pretending to myself that all was well when it wasn't, then I'd be lying to myself, which would not create dignity or kindness. The 'ists' all say that the feeling of safety grows with increased acceptance, as you meet your pain and your feelings with kindness. I was so pleased I had done that with The Boy. Instead of fearing I might be perceived as a diva or lazy or weak for allowing him to make me tea on our first date in my house, I met my own needs of physical fatigue. I could feel my body relax as it knew that it could begin to trust me. An absolute key for chronic illness recovery.

I also often reminded myself that the people I admire and love, whose stories most inspire me, are those who really GO THROUGH THINGS. I never think that someone going through darkness is weak. Quite the opposite. It breaks my heart when people who suffer from anxiety and chronic conditions perceive themselves as weak. Those with ongoing lived conditions are often the strongest, for getting up and carrying on. I nearly apologized then for being on a soapbox, but I am feeling what I am feeling and it's feeling good!

Here's a list-ette for more practical tips:

- Simply name the feelings. It's the beginning of processing them.
- Keep sharing. Or if that's too hard then . . .
- Try journalling. If I'm honest, I used to think journalling was a self-help cliché to sell more floral-patterned notebooks. It turns out, as we write our brains process our past experiences. We see the feelings and experiences as facts and not as amped-up worrying thoughts about what we are feeling. Sometimes answers can emerge as the writing stops our mind spiralling. I was firmly put in my place and now regularly write out what I am feeling.
- Sit with and allow the physical sensation of emotions without judgement. They are energy in motion and not who you are. Do ten seconds to start with before you distract. Build to a minute. Go as slowly as you like. The body prefers to let the steam out little by little.
- Have a cry for ten minutes.
- Use movement to release trapped emotion. Even when I'm unable to label exactly how I'm feeling, I

do stretches and gentle movements, like swaying or shaking things out. Slowly you'll discover the ways to release your specific emotions (e.g. a tight jaw is often due to anger). Don't forget dancing.

Do Look Back In Anger

A separate note on anger. For I personally found it one of the hardest feelings to befriend. Could I trust anger? Could I allow anger, especially when I had been led to believe it was a 'bad' emotion and ugly on a woman? I knew I had to smash that ghastly pattern. I was certainly feeling anger about my decades of misdiagnosis. Of course we can be angry at what has happened to us. Anger is often a necessary right response. Anger often needs to come before forgiveness. Without anger, little changes in the world. Without anger at suffering, compassion doesn't rise and win through. Of course we can be angry at what the world does to others. Go to the top of a hill and shout, scream into a pillow, sit in your car alone and speak it all out. Whatever you need. I was a cushion pummeller (not a euphemism). Anger frees you from the past. Bit by bit. It impassions you to move forward and make change.

I discovered that fatigue, lethargy and apathy are often the energy of trapped anger. If I let out some feelings of anger, verbally or physically (my poor cushions!), I was amazed how often my fatigue lifted. The mind–body connection was proved in an instant. I wasn't remotely scared of anger any more. I was more scared to keep it in.

Nightclubs

The other emotion the world seems to have become anxious about, in delightful irony, is anxiety. I hope it's useful to you, MDRC, to remind you that being human means we have to experience fear to survive. Part of our brain is designed to signify alert when we are in danger. Our heart rate increases and our blood flow goes to our muscles, all to give the energy and alertness to move as quickly as we can from the threat. That's the energy in motion of fear. When there is no immediate threat, and we feel those jittery sensations, that's anxiety. Just as something might anger us, our body is giving us a kindly warning signal with anxiety. I believe we can too quickly pathologize being anxious when it's not a systematic disease. Of course there are some anxiety disorders that need intervention, but if initially we can listen to the anxiety, rather than suppress it, we may be able to address what it is trying to tell us and stabilize the brain and body again.

My example of anxiety being a useful warning signal for me – and it might seem rather banal, MDRC, so bear with – was me and nightclubs at university. University life in your early twenties is obviously going to mean partying, clubbing, long nights in the pub. But many of us, sometimes unknowingly before we accepted or knew who we were, would rather pick up the runny poo of a dog belonging to another person than go clubbing. (Dog love is such that we can weirdly cope with picking up our own. To be clear, our own dog poo . . . not *our* own poo . . . why am I still typing . . . stop Miranda . . .). I like the idea of a nightclub, but one from a Hollywood classic movie with seats and tables, fantastic live music, a spot of Charleston and waiter service. Just me? The reality at uni: a long queue to buy a warm pint, being permanently too close to another human being, considerable body odour filling the air, a very sticky floor to dance to a middle-aged DJ playing the crappier eighties tunes, and men thinking they are infinitely sexier than they are as they try to shove their tongue in your mouth. You need to be very drunk to convince yourself it's fun. And I didn't drink (generally, immune system dysfunction means alcohol is not your friend). I was having a bad time the minute I walked in.

I didn't know how exhausting innocently going clubbing could make me feel. I went every week because, you know, we 'have' to go if everyone else goes, don't we? And then I started getting anxious. Because it truly went against my nature. As university years went on, I found myself getting very tired. Run-down. I didn't bounce back from a cold. I was getting more chest infections. It was harder to wake up in the mornings (and took me a good three days after a night out to recover). I was losing my energy for a lot of things I loved. A lot of that was undiagnosed Lyme disease and other viral load, but some of it was my body saying there were some anxious-making lifestyle elements which were adding stress and inflammation to my immune system. Just a simple night or two a week doing what a young person does. Harmless. We think. But I am a sit down with a few friends for a picnic, cuppa in someone's house, gentle café kind of a socializer. Big events are tiring on my system. Doing a number of activities I didn't like and my body was putting the brakes on. Those microaggressions truly do affect.

If only I had done university in the way my unique design needed to have done it. If I had understood emotional well-being like I do now, I would have sat down and talked through the feelings of anxiety to see if there was a specific cause. I may have got to the point of admitting that I didn't want to be doing politics at university at all, and I might have left to do the theatre stage management course I so longed to do. I don't know. Perhaps if I had never had a tick-borne illness, I would never have felt the effects of overdoing it from a young age. I don't know.

But I do know that anyone who goes against the grain to better serve their unique personality, who advocates for what they need, is winning.

Are you doing anything – be honest! – that you really don't like, MDRC? Are you spending time with people who make you feel stressed and drained, who go against your values? Have a little think about what you'd love to do and aren't doing . . . It might just change everything.

Can I Turn the Ship?

And yet. When you are in the middle of a bed- or housebound illness (or whatever your nightmare is at a certain time in your life, and a little hug to you if you're in it now), it is easy, I found, to wallow in what you can't do. To think of all the things you love to do that you miss. With such a long history of being unwell, it was very easy for me to dwell in the past. To wallow in my story. I knew I had to be patient because the grief, anger, disappointment and other difficult feelings post-diagnosis kept needing to be released for the full belief a new story could begin, but still I wallowed.

I wallowed and wallowed like a self-pitying hippopotamus. I splashed around in the mud and mire of unbelief, petulant that my circumstances wouldn't change, that I had lost too much time, that I had become too unwell. Oh yes, I was good at the wallowing. But here's the thing about rock-bottom: it brings with it a choice. You either stay in the mire that nothing will change, or you choose to believe that you can walk in the opposite direction. I know how lucky I am to be on the other side of it. It can take a long time to stop wallowing. And, don't tell anyone – I can still have wallow-y moments.

I was lying on my bed with the weird combination of heavy, throbbing muscular pain and a lighter, stingy hot skin, exhausted, heavy eyes and blurred vision, yet unable to sleep – oh, woe is me, the wallower. I will be honest, the effort was immense to force my mind to look in a different direction, to believe that I could have any wellness and a new beginning. It felt like my mind was the weight of a gigantic ocean liner and I had to find a way to turn 180 degrees. The weight of the past hurt. I was astounded that despite just lying there, completely still, making this mental shift felt like serious physical effort. But if it was easy, well, none of us would be in pain. Trauma wouldn't happen. Our minds would be easily trained. So there it was in all its glory. This is why we can go years without changing. This is why we remain sad and stressed and in patterns and thoughts we wish we could be without. The turning away is really hard (it's not our fault).

We want to sail on. We want to be able to turn a difficult experience around with quick positive thinking. We don't want to have to go *through* anything, thank you very much. But now I know that it is not possible without processing what's gone before.

It's a close step from wallowing to getting stuck in a sense-less WHY. Oh, goodness me, I so wanted to look up to the sky and dramatically – in full, righteous self-pity – shout a pro-longed, 'Whhhhhyyyyyyyy? Whyyyyyyyy mmeeeeeeeeee?' Especially when it briefly feels oh so good. My tippity-top tip here would be that getting stuck in 'why' really does not help. Of course we want to make sense of it. But sometimes we will never know why. There's so much of this magical, mysterious life that we will never understand.

I eventually made that mental shift from the wallowing and why-ing by, instead of demanding instant change of myself, asking myself, 'What would you do every day if you believed that you were going to be well?' Wow, that felt heavy. Heavy as in a weighty truth, because in my body I felt a lightness. I knew that was a sign of being on the right path. If I believed I could be well, I would rest, I would read when I could, I would learn all the things I know are important for well-being for my future, I would be more grateful for what I had despite confinement. I would keep practicing surrender. I would allow my feelings, I would connect more. I would think of who I was beyond illness (and I saw that was vital, whether I recovered or not).

Excitingly, this works for any situation, MDRC. It's all about seeing yourself as free from your current circumstances and taking what tiny steps you can to nurture that person that you aren't quite yet, but can be. Or more likely, know you are deep down. That wild self, that you know deserves freeing. I mean, we might as well do that?! Trust that we have a better future and start preparing for it. The alternative – the hippo. That was miserable. Of course, it's two steps forward, one back, often one forward, twenty back ... The hippo didn't immediately become a gazelle leaping about in fitness and back to work. But the hippo did float a bit more and did occasionally potter on to the banks of the river. Are you enjoying this metaphor?

Interestingly, when I did first put down the 'why me?' and turn towards a trust in a different future, there was a wave of grief. I was back in the airport baggage reclaim and could sense why at nineteen I hadn't wanted to walk back into the arrivals hall. It wasn't a safe environment to feel what I was feeling. Simply, I didn't then feel I could fully be myself. The grief was making way for a new story.

Everything Is Bigger In The Wild

When I was forced to delve into the world of well-being, I came across some seemingly peculiar suggestions and practices along the way. Some of which were very easy for me to refuse to even try and understand, like bee venom therapy – um, NO, THANKS! – or fish pedicures – STOP IT! I always need at least some science or clear foundation. Which is why I won't rush into reiki and the like. I also won't do things that are likely good for you if I simply just don't like them. Hot yoga springs to mind (the thought of holding a yoga pose in a sweat box makes me feel quite weak – I'd only go if I could sit naked in the corner with a lolly). When someone first suggested to me that I do tai chi, I launched in: 'I mean, with all respect' – by which anyone usually means no respect at all – 'it's just that kind of **** that puts everyone off trying to feel better because they see people wafting their arms about and having a green smoothie and a bit of fun and that's all very well and good if you feel okay, but when you are seriously unwell then you actually need something a bit less **** than tai ******* chi.' Though I wouldn't say this is a good example of emoting towards a fellow human just trying to make a suggestion!

And cut to me two months later in a tai chi lesson having the time of my life! I now do tai chi from time to time on my own, *often* turning it into a kind of ballet to amuse myself. (It's all about finding what works for you.) For me, tai chi revealed something very unexpected. I found doing the moves often felt awkward, especially when they require the use of one's full wingspan (not just because my wingspan is wide and I will often hit furniture or people). But it was taking up my full sense of space, of really being seen, of really being present physically that made me shy. As a performer, I was surprised by my reaction.

But it was quite the revelation. Tai chi gave me the knowledge I needed to free myself from an unhelpful childhood pattern – namely, that the younger me thought (rightly or wrongly) that she should be quieter, not disturb the peace, not ask for help, and crack on. Now, I knew that I wanted my adult/wild self to feel she could be as big as she naturally needs to be.

Rewilding

When I first went to Knepp in West Sussex, a 3,000-acre estate that has been left to rewild itself over the last twenty years, I was stunned by the effect. I walked through the gates and something instantly changed in the surroundings and in me. I felt the sense of space I had experienced in my youth when travelling (and shed a tear on realizing that truly was the last time I ever felt fit and well to live a normal life). The landscape, even a short distance from the gate, was completely different. The rewilding had created an England from 1,000 years ago, something so ancient but completely new, of course, to me. I was still in Sussex. I could sometimes hear the hum of the A24. There were oak trees and birdsong and other things I had been familiar with all my life, but it was completely different (they have storks there, for heaven's sake). I stood still, amazed. Amazed not only by the environment but by how light I felt. It's hard to explain, but at Knepp everything seemed more vibrant and alive, and I felt that in myself too.

On my first night I went for a walk at dusk. It was perhaps the first time I was in touch with a sense of us humans not being the big cheeses on this earth we think we are – if a wild, long-horned cow felt spooked and I inadvertently got between her and her calf, she might just have a go and I wouldn't have a chance. Everything around me was wild, it all felt bigger, and I felt smaller than I had before. Yet I could confidently take up my space. I was in a vast landscape that I knew I belonged in and could fit into it. No whacking of furniture if I did a tai chi move here!

Everything is bolder, brighter and more beautiful when in the wild. And once we're wild again, we're at peace. The irony is that it's often a fear of our wildness that traps us. We don't want to stand out or rock the boat. Yet it's what we must do. Don't fear your wildness. You wouldn't stop a lion from roaring, or a child from hysterically giggling, or a tree from blooming. It would be downright mean. Don't shrink to fit in, for you are loveable in your wildness.

In the dusk, it dawned on me that it keeps going back to trust in that inherent identity. Surely, if we believed we were loved fully, we would be safe to express emotions without judgement? If we could trust that we are at our most exquisite when we let ourselves go, then surely feelings would reside naturally without resistance as a glorious and intriguing part of our lives?

I was no longer going to hold it all together. Not all illnesses are caused by trapped emotion, but a lot are – it's what bodies do. They store all we experience. It's just science, and wherever you are on the spectrum from dis-ease to disease, to live fully human is to live fully present to your emotions and feelings.

I no longer feel like I'm letting myself down in previously so-called weaker emotional moments.

In fact, I feel like I have let myself up.

Second Date

Big news, MDRC, there was a second date with The Boy. I KNOW! The grumpiness of the 'pizza box shunt' did not put him off. I trusted myself to go on a second date, if nothing else to continue experimenting with not feeling small or presenting myself how I felt I 'should' rather than how and who I was. Not that he was an experiment – I wouldn't have said yes unless I genuinely liked him, I hasten to add.

He came over to have more cups of tea on my sofa (that was our only dating option still), and chatting was such that four hours felt like twenty minutes. Always a good sign. I noticed the time and found myself putting on the television and saying, 'I need to look up the tennis scores.' Please note I didn't say, like a repressed, overly apologetic woman, 'Sorry, do you mind, hope you don't think I'm rude, but is it okay if I look up the tennis scores?' I just did it. Thankfully, and of course unsurprisingly, the natural who-I-was-ness then led to discussions of all things sport and our love of watching it.

But.

Before I could switch off the TV, a news report came on to do with Covid, and it *really* irked me. I started huffing and puffing and moaning at the TV. I needed to switch it off lest I exploded. But I couldn't find the remote control. Something that really winds me up. I was so annoyed at the news footage, desperate to switch it off, I went into what looked like a full menopausal meltdown (though it was just silly old me, menopausal or not). 'Where's the remote? I just had it. Where's it gone?' He handed me one. 'NO! That's the fire stick – where's the main remote, for the television?' He handed me another one. 'NO! That's for the DVD player, which I never use, so why is that always around? The TV one. I JUST HAD IT. How can you lose something you JUST HAD?' He calmly pointed to the shelf where I had left it. 'THANK YOU,' I said crossly. Then something glorious happened. I was about to go back to old ways and apologize with a stuttering, 'Sorry, you must think I'm completely mad, I'm not normally like that, but ... so sorry ...' etc., when he giggled. And I launched into the kind of tirade normally reserved for years into married life. 'No, you are not allowed to laugh, because I was genuinely angry about that news report. It reminded me of early Covid days when the leaders were so IDIOTIC! I used to think blooming heck, get an emotionally intelligent person (i.e. a woman) up there for ten minutes a day to give a calming and clear message, and some helpful practical tips to stay emotionally healthy, and we'd be in a FAR better place. Why do leaders always have to be so emotionally averse and unintelligent?' (Yes, I know, irony.) The anger release had given me some physical energy so I was also big-time stomping. I was pacing up and down on a second date with my full wingspan flapping like a gargantuan stork in front of a shy man pinned back firmly on the sofa, slightly alarmed.

I felt sure Peggy was looking down – paws over eyes possibly, willing me on – delighted that I was with human company again, and just being the me she knew and loved unconditionally. I knew that, whatever happened with The Boy, the only way I would feel fully free and healthy would be if I allowed myself to be whole with another. No more masks!

Being angry on a second date was a good start. Plus, I was finally doing things that were casting votes for my identity beyond illness.

The Fire Pit

You see, MDRC, I hadn't realized, until Peggy died, that I had allowed my identity to become almost entirely about my health. It seemed like it was the right thing to do to start with, part of finding a solution (the opposite was true, of course). After learning what I had with this treasure, I wanted to create and mark a moment to signify my turning of the ship from the past. To celebrate being less of a wallowy old hippo! I was not yet fully healed by any stretch, but I knew it would be a step towards that hope.

I had a file full of old medical records. And a box full of old journals. I took them into the garden and got a small fire going in the fire pit. I had a brief look at some of the medical files, seeing TATT at least three times in scrawly writing. I saw endless blood test results and doctors' letters mentioning my raised inflammation levels and the constant activation of glandular fever, but reassuring me it shouldn't be a problem. Immediately I was in floods of tears over what felt like pages of lost months and years to unwellness.

I dared to peek at my journals. Some dating back to 1991. Although there were some amusing entries – particularly around a forgotten love of Jason Donovan and a strange fascination with Harold Bishop and Mrs Mangel in *Neighbours* – generally it was a repetition of why I couldn't do what everyone else

142

could, how I was going to feel better, the worry of always letting friends down, and on it went.

And on the fire it all went.

As I burned records and journals, I honoured my story with
a grief I hadn't allowed at the start. (I was veritably Spanish!)

I didn't have Peggy by my side, but because I had learnt to
allow my feelings, and watch them move through, I was able
to create a safe, loving presence for myself. I could trust
myself to look after myself with whatever life might bring.
And that brought me peace.

Treasure Four

Thoughts

TREASURES PICKED UP: Self-awareness and acceptance, mindful, connecting to your lovely body, laughter, how to rewire thoughts

PATTERNS SMASHED: Fear of stillness, separating mind and body, self-judgement and criticism, negative self-talk

WATCHWORD: Self-control

SOUNDTRACK: 'Stop! In the Name of Love' by Diana Ross and The Supremes

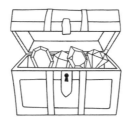

Thoughts

Home And Away

Back in 2013, a few years before the grizzly illness business had taken over my life, I was still able to work and travel. There was never a full tank of energy, and I was starting to get some more serious conditions (and injuries), but a collapse was still far off. I believe that love for my work – and the people involved – sustained me. I have a unique memory from that time, so please do leap back to 2013 with me, MDRC.

It was February and I was lying on a beach in Australia resting before a stand-up show that night. Not just any old beach but Palm Beach, where *Home and Away* was filmed, if you please! Oh yes, I had the Surf Club in eyeshot and everything. The reason it resonated so much was not just because it was the set of a TV show I used to love (clearly I had a minor obsession with Australian soaps . . .), but because I was lying on the *exact* spot I had been twenty-one years before, when I was on my travelling adventure. Everything was the same – the timeless waves, the offshore breeze, the almost-orange sand, the grassy banks above the beach, the scorching Australian sun, and even the trailers, vans and crew members indicating that *Home and Away* was still filming. Even – wait for it (for those who know) – the actor who played Alf! (Maybe it was a major obsession. Let's not dwell.)

There I was, everything the same – except, of course, what twenty-one years of life does to a person. The experiences it adds, the suffering it takes, the dreams it fulfils, the unmet dreams it neglects, the wisdom gained, the innocence lost. Despite all the changes, I felt in many ways, at my core, the same. I know now that our core self – that wild, natural person with our unique personalities, skills and traits – is a constant. Yet it becomes buried by roles, responsibilities and those so-called worldly rules in adulthood. Sitting on that beach, I palpably felt the link to so many aspects of the freer nineteen-year-old me I was longing to express again.

Aged nineteen on Palm Beach, I was as an athlete, lean and fit. I was a dreamer but very much in the moment, exploring, interested, expressive. I was loud when I wanted to be, quiet when I needed to be. I was adventurous – we took the dramatic route and flew to Cairns from Sydney, then headed into the outback by bus and made our way down the sparsely populated West Coast. I was unbound from the need for a clear path or career to follow. I was unbound from needing to wear make-up or fit into a fashion or dress code, and I was unbound from having a diary full of social obligations. I was doing all the things I loved – I didn't have to search for hobbies. I lived off Vegemite sandwiches due to budgetary constrictions, but didn't feel I lacked a thing. Ditto sharing dorms in youth hostels or sleeping under corrugated-iron-roofed sheds next to service stations in the outback. I slept well. Inadvertently, I was doing all that I needed to do to live healthily – in purpose, in connection, in the moment, inspired and excited, joyful and playful, exercising just by the nature of what I was loving to do each day. I was not swayed by decisions or choices that didn't align with my values.

Today, I am grateful for the understanding that these are vital lessons for how I *always* need to be. I still feel a familiar twinge of sadness when I recall that nineteen-year-old self, landing back at Heathrow airport after her travels, and how pressured she felt to be and do in ways other than her honest self, to live a so-called 'successful life'.

However free I was in my youth, let's not paint an untrue rose-tinted picture. By nature of being a human with a mind, I did of course, like all teenagers, have worries. Sitting in that exact same spot above the beach twenty-one years earlier gave me an intriguing opportunity to reflect on them. My 1992 top-line worries were:

- What if I get bitten by a funnel-web spider?
- I want to ask to be an extra on *Home and Away*, but I might embarrass myself.
- I don't think I can tell anyone back home that I want to be an actress; they might persuade me against my dream.
- I wonder if I will ever like big parties. Do I have to like big parties?
- Am I weird?
- If I am weird, is it because I'm long and gangly?
- Someone said they once saw a funnel-web spider in their breakfast cereal cupboard in central Sydney. I'm going to check under the pillows tonight.

149

- What happens if my appendix bursts when we are in the middle of the outback?
- I hope I earn money to travel when I am older.
- I hope I make friends with some creative people so I can be silly with them.
- It's so spooky that humans can live in a big city among tiny spiders that can actually kill them.
- I hope I don't put on weight, though if I do, I might be less gangly and goofy.
- I hope it's okay that I really don't want to snog anyone in a youth hostel. I only want to be with someone I know and like well.
- What happens if I get bitten by a funnel-web and get appendicitis at the same time and they only treat one and I die of the other?

I have written myself a reply.

Ah, little one, dear girl, bless you. Firstly, can I just say you were so incredibly brave to do all that travelling. With no phone. And with the constant threat of death by funnel-web spider or appendicitis. I'm not laughing at you – and would like to share that in the twenty-one years since then, I have never been bitten by a spider or had an emergency operation. And also, guess what: you became an actress. It took you a few more years to tell anyone, but you worked hard, and you did it. You have silly creative friends with whom you make up dance routines and sing randomly and wander around without a bra on and they care not. And I don't want to scare you, but the acting thing went quite, well, explosive. You ended up becoming a bit famous. Don't worry – your shyness left you, and you took it all with a pinch of salt and enjoyed the ride.

Oh, and guess what, we just had lunch in a café near the *Home and Away* filming (yes, they're still going) and sat with fans of a show you wrote (long story). The fans were joking that I should ask for a part in *Home and Away*! I feel I let you down by not asking. But look, you're in Australia, so you managed to travel again. And I want to tell you the biggest thing – you are not and never were weird. You are not even gangly (someone just said that to you once in the playground and it stuck in your head). You have a figure to die for and it's absolutely okay that you are not ready for a boy to get anywhere near it.

Oh, and no, you will never like big parties and that's also more than okay. I am just so sorry that you never felt it was okay. I should warn you some dreams didn't come true. You don't have chickens or donkeys. You haven't done a duet with Jason Donovan. And you didn't become a secretary in the Foreign Office to travel for a living. But there are some dreams that were never meant to come true (the latter being an excellent example). But, my dear beautiful girl, all is well with you. There are some difficulties, there are some remnants of worries that will perhaps always be with us, but all is well. Do you remember those two quotes we had on our bedroom wall?

'I've lived through some terrible things in my life, some of which actually happened.' – Mark Twain

' "Supposing a tree fell down, Pooh, when we were underneath it?"

"Supposing it didn't," said Pooh after careful thought. Piglet was comforted by this.' – A. A. Milne

I will make you a promise that I will do my very best to keep your wild, free self front and centre, because I wish you had been taught to trust your instincts and told how great you intrinsically were, so you didn't have half those worries. I love you, you gangly weirdo. Too soon?!

At Home With Thoughts

It was a delightful distraction from the dark cave of illness to be back in the sun and sand and space of Australia (in my mind). And also delightful that I knew nineteen-year-old me would agree with me now, that our greatest dream is to be at home with our thoughts, free and confident in our own skin. Isn't that everyone's dream, really?

This then galvanized me, MDRC, to wake up to any thoughts that might be driving current suffering (plus I didn't want to have another list of unnecessary worries I could write myself in twenty-one years' time). I knew already, from the 'ists', that it's often the thoughts *about* circumstances that cause the most suffering, rather than the circumstances themselves. To that end, I considered that thoughts might be similar to the effects of emotions on the body. Certainly, by continuing to surrender to symptoms, and acknowledging my feelings about the condition I was living with, I was sustaining some physical improvement. I was prepared to dig and delve further, in the hope of finding more treasures about the mind–body connection. To heal.

In your face, Lyme disease and your ghastly associated conditions!

What Are Thoughts?

MDRC, we are so lucky to live at a time when cutting-edge neuroscience shows what spiritual wisdom and teachings have told us through the ages. We now know – and it's MIND-BLOWING, MDRC (pun absolutely intended, and I doubt it will be the last time I use it) – that thoughts are *actual* matter. They are made of proteins and chemicals. Yes, our thoughts are actual *things*. So, if we repeatedly align with negative thoughts, they will strengthen, form a long-term memory and lead to a toxic-stress response. Basically, what we think about actually grows. MIND-BLOWING. Every bit of our brain chemistry affects every cell in our body, so that if we are in toxic stress, from the negative thoughts, it can lead to pain, inflammation and disease. Wow.

We also now know that the mind is separate from the brain. Whaaaat?! MIND-BLOWING. So that means it's our mind – i.e. our will, choices, habits, every thought – that affects our brain. The thoughts we have either grow good, healthy, nourishing trees in our brain or they don't. And our brain is the powerhouse of the body where the immune system, nervous system and hormonal system are housed. Without a healthy brain we cannot have a healthy body. Therefore, as all the 'ists' tell us, it is unsound and scientifi-cally impossible to separate mind and body.

Wow again. So every fear or irritation towards my physical

condition was worsening it. Even perhaps, for all I knew, a reason it was being perpetuated. This was already a sparkling treasure from the cave wall.

I was relieved to hear that thoughts are not inherently bad. We're always going to have them. Many of them are good as we need to plan, rationalize, trouble-shoot, invent, search for genuine threats. And the negative ones are harmless if we let them fly in and out without attachment. Then they simply flit away before they can form a lasting thought tree (or neural pathway). It's only when we believe and invest in thoughts over and over again that they become a strong pathway, eventually forming a belief to live by and operate from. (These beliefs can of course be negative or positive, unhealthy or healthy.)

And thrice wow. For that means subconscious negative beliefs could have been diluting my wild self. Oh, I was going to have no more of that, thank you very much. I did not want to operate under any kind of fear, certainly not unknowingly. I was galvanized further.

I found this incredibly helpful quote from Buddhist teacher Yongey Mingyur Rinpoche in his book *In Love with the World*: 'The less we know about the chattering, muttering voice in our head that tells us what to do, what to believe, what to buy, which people we should love, and so forth, the more power we grant it to boss us around and convince us that whatever it says is true.'

And a fourth wow to that, for I want to be the boss! I didn't want any toxic negative protein trees in my brain thank you very much please. This too showed me the importance of surrender, for without facing difficult thoughts – and hearing them – I wouldn't have known what I needed to change.

There's One Good Plastic In This World!

MDRC, we're ever luckier to know from the 'ists' that we can change our brains. Our brains are plastic. We can rewire and grow healthier trees and kill off the toxic ones. THANK GOD!

Say it with me, children: What's the good plastic? That's it – neuroplastic!

I hope that schools soon have a full curriculum on emotional well-being so that we can teach young humans how to human a bit better. I definitely would have had an easier existence had I been taught in at least one science lesson that if I was feeling under the weather or sad or anxious, it might be because I was thinking negative thoughts, which all minds do, which in turn create some toxic reactions, a bit like eating poison. And I could choose to put something sweeter and kinder in my mind to make me feel better. You can take your periodic tables and your Bunsen burners; I needed *that*. (I really hope young people are no longer frightened into thinking they are ill or weird for feeling normal human emotions and thoughts. For that was occasionally the case in my youth, for sure.)

Our brains can change. They are highly adaptable. We can think in new ways. Whatever thoughts we repeat most often, we reinforce and build new neural pathways. Whatever thoughts we don't use or reinforce will grow weak and eventually fade away. THANK GOD!

I may not have had a crystal ball to peer into my future and the degree of wellness yet to come, but I knew that changing the thinking response to my condition was the only way I would have a chance to get well. I was teary-eyed with relief that there was something I could do. Especially in the phases I was still confined to bed.

It was time to find the practices for this theory and be the boss of my brain.

Self-Control

I'm not a stoic. I prefer the gentlest of approaches to pretty much anything. If anything feels pushed, I wobble. But steady yourself, MDRC, for I'm going to quote a stoic at your lovely face!

> 'You have power over your mind – not outside events. Realize this, and you will find strength . . . Our life is what our thoughts make it.'
> – Marcus Aurelius

The word self-control kept coming to mind. I know, it doesn't seem like a very contemporary word or stance. Nor particularly friendly for this sensitive soul. I looked up the meaning – the ability to regulate and restrain one's thoughts, emotions and behaviours in the face of trials. Yup, my instinct was right, that was what I needed. Self-control became my watchword for this treasure.

I had a moment of understanding that our great baby-boomer (and indeed older) generation(s) might reasonably question our

156

focus on emotional well-being, and likely think we often should buck up and stop feeling, processing and assessing. That generation knows only too well, there will be times we need to find strength and control to carry on even if we feel we can't. But, I believe, we need both. We need the resilience to keep going, knowing that we won't crumble in a heap inappropriately. No one wants an inappropriate crumble! And we need to know that we have the permission to crumble, unafraid of our thoughts and emotions, when we can't be effective until they have moved through us or we have addressed the issue.

At this stage in my recovery, I needed to find some discipline for what I was learning. I was still housebound but the release of grief and expressing anger had created a little more brain energy to focus. It was time for a gentle nudge into self-control (not a 'button up and push on' moment), to put some daily practices into place that would help me uncover any subconscious beliefs that might be affecting my physiology.

I thought about The Boy – The Boy from Bristol as I started to call him (because he was from Bristol; I know, I am soooo clever) – and how a romantic relationship could be a distraction from my studies. The most important relationship right now, I knew, was with myself as I kept walking towards that new version of me at the end of the cave I hoped to meet. New, but similar, as I picked up the hidden wild parts of my nineteen-year-old self I missed and needed.

I wondered. Might these treasures, perhaps, be in some ways a love letter to that younger self?

Top Ten Tunes

Before we can change our thoughts, we first need to become conscious of the ones that cause us angst. Our 'top ten tunes' (a term used by expert life-coach sociologist, and all-round lovely person Martha Beck). These are different for everyone, but I found it reassuring to learn that up to 90 per cent of our thoughts are repeated, the same old tunes played over and over. On the advice of the 'ists', I regularly took a few moments throughout the day to acknowledge what I was thinking and feeling, writing down the headline thoughts that made me feel miserable or stressed. It only took a couple of weeks to see what my top ten tunes were. The playlist of my mind.

Unsurprisingly, at that time most of my top ten tunes were focused on my health. With all that I had lost from illness, there was distinct fear around never getting better. 'I will never get better' was certainly a top five thought, along with 'my body is too worn down now'. Oh, and the ghastly 'it's all my fault I am so sick.' RUDE! It's a testament to the ability to rewire the brain that I can't now remember the other top ten tunes of the time. I think they included the good old 'I'm wasting my time' – she always likes to be heard! Most people, I understand, have some version of 'I'm not good enough' as their number one (that hurts my heart). Mine has been *it's* not good enough', about circumstances. Surrendering and looking for the good in the moment was always hard when that thought was active.

We need a lot of self-control to not get stuck in our habitual patterns of thought. Especially when they feel so true and have been such a big part of our subconscious. Yet there's no one else who can be accountable for our thoughts, as no one else knows them. I don't think there can be a much better use of our time than to rewire our minds, can there? And if negative thoughts affect our brain, which affects our body, it will lead to good health too. Why didn't I learn this at school? I mean, I have *yet* to use a Bunsen burner in adulthood . . . or a protractor . . . or Latin . . . (Keep studying, kids, you never know what your unique life skill will need!)

The Five Whys

Another Martha Beck tool I found useful when trying to uncover deep-rooted thoughts is 'The Five Whys'. You name the thought you want to address and then question it with a 'why', then ask 'why?' to the answer and keep going until you invariably find a 'why' you can't answer. At that point, you'll have likely found the root of your fearful thought. I first tried this on a particularly bad day, when I didn't have enough energy to go downstairs. The walls of my bedroom were closing in on me and I noticed a top five tune barging unhelpfully into my mind:

I am so desperate to get better so that I can work and travel again.

Why, Miranda?

Well, whoever it is that I am currently talking to (this is a bit odd, but I'll go with it), *because then I can have fun and great experiences and achieve things.*

159

Why do you need to do those things?

I suppose because then I justify life. Life isn't a dress rehearsal and all that . . .

Why do you need to justify life?

Um, because . . . then I haven't wasted time or my existence.

Why do you need to prove you have not wasted your existence?

Ummm. (I was getting somewhere. This was harder to answer.) *I have to prove with doing because, ummm . . .*

Yes? Why?

Because otherwise what's the point in my life?

I gasped. Did I really just say that? *What's the point in my life?* That felt like one step away from '*What's the point in me?*' And I know that to be nonsense because there's a point in all of us – we are each inherently loved and valued. I certainly did not want that pesky thought flying about. Nor did I want the one about my life not having a point unless it was justified through productivity and experiences. I would never say that to another person – loved one or stranger. Yet there it was. A part of me was so conditioned to believe that the point of me was solely to be productive that I couldn't separate achievement from a good life.

160

With a root thought like 'What's the point in my life?', it can lead to a limiting belief I understand many people have – 'I have not done enough.' Doing over being. That would be why I used to push my body, and why I fought against an illness that wasn't my fault. There is a very damaging cycle people can get caught up in – the boom and bust it's called. Pushing for productivity when feeling energetic enough and then crashing and burning with the overdoing. Those with ME and chronic fatigue syndrome (CFS) will know it well. The crash being our bodies putting the brakes on and saying the pace is too much. The world's trajectory of productivity and/or seeking wealth, status and comfort means we have exploded internally, burning out inside to seek the outside. It was a huge relief for it to sink in head to heart once and for all, that the external can't make me happy. There is a point in me and my life, even when I am, or remain, sick.

It was a blessing in heavy disguise to discover all this, but I was excited, MDRC. When we become conscious of the patterns that keep us spinning, we can change. There is hope.

You Are A Lot Nicer Than You Think You Are!

The hardest part of looking under the hood at our thoughts is to face and understand our inner critic. We all have one. The inner critic is the bully that says things like, 'I can't believe you said that at the party, you're an idiot.' And that's her on a good day. The inner critic will be the one saying you aren't strong enough, funny enough, beautiful enough, achieving enough – the one with the meanest thoughts, constantly saying you should be better in some way or other.

One of my favourite sayings I discovered when studying surrender was 'Rest is to be, without reporting on being.' So often, unknowingly, we're judging ourselves and reporting our failures: 'You didn't do that well enough, oh you made a mistake there, you're not as good as anyone else, you'll always fail in some way, you shouldn't be crying, you should be over this illness by now.' ('Shoulds' always usually equals shame.) I don't think it's too harsh to say that we abuse ourselves internally when judging in that way. Our wild selves become completely beaten down under such a critical regime.

I'm pleased to say that there is absolutely no reason to beat ourselves up about the inner critic's existence. (That would be a ghastly loop if we were criticising ourselves for having an inner critic.) It's part of the protective mechanisms of childhood. Remember, part of our survival was the need to belong to our caregiver. If we had a caregiver who, for example, kept telling us to be quiet and pipe down, it can turn inwards, becoming an inner critic thought like, *Oh, I'm just too much.* The inner critic was trying to help us to belong. But now we need to understand that it isn't needed any more.

A friend told me she was on a date and when she naturally did a massive, over-the-top laugh, a thought from her past popped in: *Oops, that laugh was too loud and silly.* She began policing herself for the rest of the meal and her natural spark was dimmed. A feeling of embarrassment or shame can ruin a moment when, the truth is, you are beautiful and brilliant and you can laugh as loudly and ridiculously as you like. I

162

know a lot of people fear their loud laughs, their snorts and guffaws – I have an amusing opposite with a silent wheeze and a wide, gummy grin, and until you know me you don't know quite what's happening!

(And the world itself is a critic. Look this way, act this way, do this to be successful, you need to have a million followers. No wonder we end up judging ourselves.)

The holy grail is to calmly see the thoughts, befriend and thank the inner critic for having helped us survive, and rewire away knowing the thoughts are not who we are. It's amazing that it's possible to quieten a harsh inner critic so we no longer have to live under their rule, and can start to flourish. Good word, FLOURISH.

Because remember, MDRC, if we start living by core negative beliefs – like 'there's no point in me' or 'I'm not good enough' – that will be the mentality we operate from. Our whole life, behavioural patterns, fears and moods are dictated by our core beliefs. MIND-BLOWING. If we believe we can't trust people, then we may be scared to have relationships and put up a guard. Anxious people start to see the danger everywhere, angry people think of all the ways they have been hurt. If I continued to believe I would never get well, I would have stayed in a ball in my bed. Basically, we *always* find proof for what we believe.

Here's what to believe, because it's true: you are a lot nicer than you think you are. You are that perfect unique majestic elephant, and you deserve to be uncaged, free from thoughts that say anything differently.

I'm very happy to be a broken record – there's only one of you. There is no one like you that has come before, and no one will do so after you are gone. You are therefore genuinely uniquely extraordinary and valuable.

Our Lovely Bodies

So here I was, MDRC – all revved up for some practical tools to make changes (as revved up as a middle-aged woman in a long fluffy dressing gown on her sofa gets). But reflecting on the truth that there's only one of me, I was first given the chance to face another limiting belief head-on. The good old 'I am not attractive' one. All the little jibes from others or the inner critic had built up over the years into a belief that I was someone for whom it wasn't acceptable to be beautiful or sexy.

There's another familiar twinge of sadness when I see that even when I was beautifully young and lean (and could easily have been a beach babe extra on *Home and Away*), I worried and complained about my body aesthetically. I hear almost every woman over forty say the same. I mean, if I am very honest with you, MDRC, I had a stereotypical supermodel physique in my youth that I would often get spotted to be a catwalk model. I couldn't walk down fashion central King's Road in London without some shop or brand shoving me their card. Yet, with this silly belief in my brain unknowingly running the show, I wouldn't tell anyone, and I'd throw the cards away. And when my body gained a considerable amount of weight in my late twenties, I felt shame rather than the self-compassion I would show it now for it being a part of my life story.

Luckily, I was eventually able to change this limiting belief quite quickly. All hail neuroplasticity! I simply started to take on board that there was no one else who looked like me and slowly but surely fell in love with what I looked like and made friends with my body. I created a new pathway in my brain that grew the positive belief that I was attractive. There's only one of me, and therefore I am uniquely beautiful. Deal with it, world . . . I'm FLOURISHING!

Interestingly, when I was getting to know The Boy from Bristol, I was able to be angry and weepy, but the thought of being naked . . . oh gosh, help, heavens! Despite the rewiring, an old kernel flagged up (not a euphemism – we're in dangerous territory). Having lost fitness due to illness, the old belief that I wasn't good enough in the sexy, womanly department returned. There were the inevitable amusing discussions with friends about meeting people later in life, when things are naturally floppier and flabbier (*Floppier and Flabbier* – a possible title for my next book). I didn't know whether the loss of my perfect companion in Peggy would be replaced by another dog, or a man, or both, but I knew there was a next level of befriending of my physical appearance needed. I didn't want to take myself out of the love game because of fearful limiting beliefs, especially as, I don't mind saying, MDRC, I was becoming more and more intrigued by The Boy from Bristol. I refocused on my authentic belief on the matter – that our bodies are a key part of us, but not the most important part. Our bodies don't define who we are. As my body changes – *Floppier and Flabbier: The Return*, followed by *The Revenge of Floppy and Flabby* – my person (if I found him), wouldn't love me less.

More importantly, our body is a finely attuned piece of intelligent equipment to help us live our life and give us life, yet so often it gets shouted at if it's not conforming to our ideal. We can't come home to ourselves if we hate the body we have been given to live in. That's when a detachment from our body can begin and it's easy to numb out, eat badly, not notice or accept how it's feeling, get injured and more. We owe it to our health to befriend our lovely bodies.

Oh, and get this heavy revvy – our bodies can't lie. Look at what you do every day, what makes your body stressed and what makes your body relax and feel excited. If we're constantly making choices out of fear, or 'shoulds' and 'musts', our bodies weaken. All those micro lies in the way we live literally affect our physiology. MIND-BLOWING.

Our dear bodies are simply trying to keep balanced and heal themselves. They are entirely efficient, intelligent, kind and resourceful. I am forever grateful to have learnt that our thoughts can get in the way of that process. I believed it was solely my body that was the problem when I became ill. I was angry at it. It was time to partner with it, disrupt old beliefs, keep learning to accept and surrender to it so as to learn what it needs to heal.

I knew that the dream of having a still mind and being at home in myself was not a childish, elusive desire, but the way to be healthy.

Retreats And Mindfulness

As I moved into the practical ways to rewire my thoughts, I was struck by how many times in the past I had tried to find some peace of mind externally. I clearly knew on some level I needed to slow the whirring pace of my thoughts and do something about how stressed I often was; but without the tools I gathered in the cave, I must have felt at a loss of what to do for permanent change.

The thought of a spa I always found reassuring. Lounging in warm rooms that mimic an exotic clime, swimming, a sauna. Delicious. But if I did go on a spa retreat, the effect would usually only last a day or two. And, on reflection, the whole experience is never entirely relaxing. Jacuzzis, for example. They're a bit strange. Sitting in hot, bubbling water, our sweat merging with strangers whom we don't know whether to smile at with a polite 'hello to you and thanks for sharing this moment with me' or avoid eye contact with at all costs. I always seemed to suffer from the awkwardness of the bust zone of my swimming costume inflating with the bubbles, and I couldn't decide whether to keep pushing it down and moving position to release the air (for fear the noise would be miscon-strued) or let it be. Let people decide if it was my flesh or inflating fabric. Once, it inflated so much that it became like a buoyancy aid, and I ended up floating about banging into people's knees!

Mindfulness was a practical tool I always felt I should try. But just the notion unnerved me. (Now, I would clock the 'I *should* try it', knowing a 'should' rarely means something truthful to do.) As the saying goes, if you haven't suffered, you haven't got still. Even adrenalin junkies and adventurers admit the hardest thing is to sit still. If I ever tried mindfulness in the past, simply knowing the basics – to watch my thoughts come and go without judgement – then ten minutes felt like about forty-five days. Plus, I was worried if I showed an interest, I might be forced to sit awkwardly on a bed of quinoa in a yoga studio for an hour with a headband made of crispy kale. Or something!

I am not laughing at mindfulness experts, it's another game-changer at the right time. If you can regularly observe your thoughts, you can slowly see that you are not your thoughts. And that can really free us. But when I was seriously ill, it was too much too soon to sit still with my mind.

For me the first step was distraction. Even distracting for a few minutes helps lower cortisol caused by fearful thoughts and shows the brain we're going in a new way. It wasn't avoidant distracting – I wasn't numbing out. To rewire it needs to be intentional. Just for a couple of minutes I would notice the scary thoughts or feelings and say 'It's okay' (even if I didn't believe it yet) and then do some kind of gentle activity or distraction. Lego, slow movement, naming things I saw out of the window, looking at colours in the room that I liked, learning something new – Duolingo, anyone? I got in touch with my senses and looked for what I could touch, taste, hear, see and smell – a great hack to get out of the whirring mind (and why music and nature are so helpful). I've heard some brain retraining experts call it looking for the 'glimmers'. Instead of focusing on triggers, look for things that make you feel cheerful or peaceful. I love that – let's get glimmering, MDRC.

168

Whenever I do, I see clearly that reality is always kinder than my thoughts.

My confinement meant I couldn't go to a spa or try a meditation or yoga class, or any of the ways we try and retreat. My bed was my retreat. It was often scary, not having the ability to escape. But it gave me the gift of time to focus on key neuroscientific practices to change my mind and the way it was operating.

I'm not against going back to a lovely spa hotel if I should be so lucky (I need to master the art of communal jacuzzi if nothing else), but I'm grateful I no longer crave such comfort and adventure to escape from myself.

Choose A New Thought

As I write, the Queen of Rock and Roll, Tina Turner, has just died. I was very moved by her death as I'd recently watched a documentary about her and had previously no idea quite how severe the domestic abuse she'd gone through was, let alone the other pressures and sadnesses in her life. I came across a quote by her: 'If a negative thought arose, I would repeat a positive one eight times in a row to counteract it. Soon, I began loving myself, imperfections and all. I stopped comparing myself to others and at last I started to look good to myself.' Her core belief, due to abuse, had become that she was not good enough for relationships. But by choosing and repeating a new thought, over and over, she could feel the change. Once you have identified your top ten tunes, you can start to tune in and sing the opposite.

Here is one of the best ways to start doing that, from the fascinating Byron Katie who I quoted in Treasure Two; I note that many other 'ists' are using this too. She calls it 'The Work', but for simplicity's sake I call it 'The Five Questions', because it's five questions (I know, I'm a bit of a genius). You start with a difficult or negative thought like 'I will never get better'. And you pose five questions to see if they may dismantle it.

1. **Can you know that that is true?** (Usually I'd answer an immediate yes to that, so scared was I about not getting better. Which is why her second question is so clever.)
2. **Can you absolutely know that that is true?** (Okay, in this instance, I'll admit no.)
3. **Who are you with that thought?** (She suggests listing all the feelings, behaviours or moods you have with that thought. I was scared, confused, helpless, and felt trapped.)
4. **Who are you without that thought?** (Imagine how you would feel without that thought existing. It can take a beat, particularly if it's a nasty firmly rooted familiar thought pattern. I sensed a lightening. Without that thought, I would feel lighter, more peaceful, accepting and self-compassionate.)
5. **What is an alternative to that thought?** (If you have felt better without the thought, then think of alternatives that feel peaceful, accepting and self-compassionate.)

Well, Miranda, I chatted to myself, if I chose the thought 'I might get better', how would that change things? I felt a peace about where I was, even though I was severely limited physically. I felt like I was in my life and not waiting for it to start. I was more surrendered. There was room for self-compassion instead of an accompanying sense that I or life had let me down. I tested the 'ists' – I meditated back on 'I will never get better'. There was an instant tightening and adrenalin shot. Wow, this just got real! Thoughts really can make you feel and stay ill. Actual and literal fact. But also – vice versa. Yay! Whenever you find yourself believing a statement is true that makes you feel bad in any way, identify ways that the opposite could also be true. It was worth every moment of diving for the self-control to go a new way.

'Stop! In The Name Of Love'

As music is known to be such a great distraction for the brain, this is the hack I use to rewire. If I notice thoughts I don't want to be a part of my life, I speak or sing 'Stop! In the Name of Love' by The Supremes. Let me explain!

STOP! This works because we need to do something definite to interrupt the old whirring stories. I will often put up my hands too, to make my brain pay attention. Do a little move, feel a bit pop-starry (which comes naturally to me, obvs . . .). Then I say or sing:

IN THE NAME OF LOVE. This tells me to take a deep breath, smile and cross my arms over to hold the opposite arm. The 'ists' say those things signal safety to the body. Which in turn gives the mind space to drop the negative story. Next it's . . .

BEFORE YOU BREAK MY HEART. This reminds me that any negative, shaming or critical thoughts that might be at play can literally hurt my heart. I remind myself I am dignified just by being (I mean, I just did a mighty pop star pose if nothing else . . .) and I don't deserve cruel internal criticism. Neither do you, MDRC. Finally . . .

THINK IT OVER. The final line of this joyful refrain tells me to choose the healthier thought, over and over. Then it's time to move intentionally on to something fun and distracting, to stop the old ways trying to sneak back in. Always try and follow the joyful glimmers. Hark at us, FLOURISHING (I'll stop using that word now . . .).

'Laughter Really Is The Best Medicine'

I wonder if the phrase 'laughter is the best medicine' originates from the biblical proverb 'a joyful heart is good medicine'. Wherever it hails from, on an experiential level, it feels true. The energy and life I feel from even a little laugh is undeniable. Now we are so very clever, MDRC, and know that thoughts are proteins and can be toxic or the opposite; well, laughter is the greatest opposite and is *literally* 'good medicine'. If you are able to treat your fears lightly, the brain stops perceiving them as a threat and your system can calm and reduce stress and anxiety.

It can be the perfect tool to use at times. I have a friend with whom I call some habitual thoughts that have become fears a 'serious threat'. They of course aren't, but our minds try to convince us they are (like the funnel-web spiders stuck in cereal boxes in Sydney!), so by going into a comedic dramatic language, like a severe newsreader, of 'this is a serious threat', my friend and I found we couldn't help but laugh at them.

We may not use this on an extremely troubling top ten tune when in a dark patch, but occassionally we have experimented. I will never forget the day we first tried it out.

We decided to go canoeing in a two-person canoe. My friend was fairly scared of the concept of going in a canoe full stop – the capsize threat, the physical strength needed, the fact that we were canoeing on a murky tidal river which she really didn't want to fall into especially as the tide might carry us downstream and out to sea (I know I have history here – this was years before my sinking mud experience!). I was already laughing at her fears. Not unkindly, just in that we were already proving the point to ourselves how 'silly' our thoughts can be. I reassured her that we would be safe and she knew she'd regret not going on a tranquil potter along an English river on a beautiful hot summer day. But by mentioning the heat (and it was very hot), it was my turn to panic a little. I have had a fear of fainting since I was a child. I started saying, 'The serious threat is of course we get heat stroke and faint.' She laughed. She thought I was joking. More evidence that my fainting fear was just a habitual pattern, it's not a serious threat – as she pointed out, we aren't constantly walking over bodies of people who have fainted in the street! We were pretty giggly at this stage because she was then worrying that if I did faint, she might not be able to control the boat, and we'd capsize and be swept away. And I was then worried that we might imbibe some of the water that would no doubt lead to some severe gastro disease! On the amusement went of analysing our different fearful thoughts that the other couldn't understand. Inadvertent therapy via canoeing.

Eventually, we set off. And all was idyllic. Although I was glad I had a large hat as the fear of sunstroke was still around (SERIOUS THREAT!). I was distracted as my friend started warbling, 'Oh no, oh no, oh no. No, really, this *is* a serious threat.' I asked her what was. The answer that came back was, 'That swan.' I unsuccessfully tried to hide my giggles. She said, 'No, seriously, this is a serious threat, seriously.' She told me if we got in the swans' waters, they might attack us, and they're strong enough to break a human's neck. I told her I thought it was an arm not a neck, but either way it wasn't a serious threat. If it was, there would be signs on the river-banks. Much as people aren't constantly fainting in the streets, nor are there hourly attacks on humans by deathly swans!

We laughed and she bravely sojourned up-river, passing the swan who of course barely glanced our way. We were back to idyllic riverbank life – albeit me swigging unnecessary amounts of water (and wondering if I should have electrolytes and a banana) and her doing a small scream if the canoe even rocked the tiniest amount!

After an hour or so it was genuinely getting very hot and we felt it would be sensible to turn around with the tide, so we didn't have to do so much paddling, head back and get into the shade. We made a rash decision to take a shortcut back, through a tributary.

We started paddling and it was getting narrower, more overgrown and harder to get through. I was sweating in the high-noon sun, and beginning to get a bit anxious. My friend was giggling at me. And then – and this is as if God planted it to give us a wonderful lesson, I jest you not – we found ourselves SURROUNDED BY SWANS. We had come up against some nests, some broods, and there were about six very large swans approaching and surrounding us. I mean, even I thought it felt a little threatening.

The only answer was to turn around – we weren't going to get through this tiny rivulet anyway. But you try turning around a ten-foot canoe in a ten-foot-wide river while surrounded by six angry hissing swans! We were in a mix of blind panic and absolute hysteria because here we were under SERIOUS THREAT!!!

Of course we got out unscathed, with no death by swan, no fainting, and the canoe and our minds eventually floated downstream as we focused on the beauty of the surrounds and the metaphor.

I love the fact that if we begin to share our fears, however absurd they may or may not be, two things happen. Not only do said fears disperse more readily, we are also able to see that our friends' fears are different to our own. We prove those fears really are just habits particular to us, rather than some universal truth. Dare to share your worries (however ridiculous), I say.

A Big Word On Little Words And Their Impact

Here's the final nugget I want to impart to you, MDRC, from this treasure – I found it incredibly important in helping to treat my condition. I hope it might help whatever you could be going through, as I think that it can be applied to anything. Get this, the words we speak have a profound effect on our well-being. Our brains hear everything we say, and if we're constantly repeating a story like 'I am so exhausted' our physiology will respond and it will affect our mood and behaviour. MIND-BLOWING! The number of times I would say things like, 'It's like wading through treacle,' or, 'It's such a battle.' Now, phrases like that make me feel instantly weak.

I had to take certain words out of my lexicon for my recovery. Eventually I stopped saying Lyme or any of the other diagnostic words, because each time I did it spooked me. I also stopped saying '*my* fatigue' or '*my* pain' so to, as it were, reduce its power. In fact, I even changed the names in case I needed to communicate to loved ones – fatigue became leaping gazelle (something to the opposite), Lyme disease become Melon and so on. (I was right about changing disease names.) There truly is power in words. I'm pretty sure not many of us get away with not having been damaged by some words spoken over us in our formative years.

And never forget the little big word: YET. If it's true that how we talk about ourselves to ourselves can determine our experience, then instead of saying, 'I can't do X,' try 'I'm not good at X . . . YET.' Down with the inner critic!

I keep saying, 'I'm not head of the Olympics ... yet,' as a controlled experiment. So, watch out ... there will be the 100m gallop, the 200m space hopper, and over-fifties trampolining. And that's just for starters ...

I came back to my watchword for this treasure – self-control. From disciplining myself to question my thoughts and find more peaceful alternatives, to 'stopping in the name of love', to using music and nature and my senses as distraction, to changing my language to be kinder, I slowly started to recover.

The hope is there. Thankfully so, because I'll be honest, MDRC, I've had a shitty few days. I know, hark at me sharing and showing off I can do vulnerable! I have been sleeping badly, I have a distractedly tight neck and sore head, and I have restless leg syndrome (a frantically irritating symptom from years ago – and hello to you if you are in the restless leg camp – imagine a camp for people with restless legs, what a bizarre leg-flailing cult it would appear . . .). My body was telling me something, and instead of ignoring it as I would have in the past, I listened to the thoughts around it. I could hear an old tune shouting loudly, 'God, it's annoying to feel like this, it ruins my fun and my life.' Just noticing that thought and I felt stressed. I closed my eyes, took five slow, deep breaths and asked myself how I was really feeling.

I was frustrated and impatient, and had some fear that my illness could return in force. Ah, there it was. Some symptoms had triggered that old fearful tune of never getting better. I allowed the feelings, had a little weep and my body loosened its grip. I opened my eyes. My mind was already calmer. I said to myself out loud, 'I might get better.' And I smiled.

Treasure Five

Loving Ourselves

TREASURES PICKED UP: Self-compassion, self-esteem, forgiving of others, clarity, authenticity, asking for help, boundaries, trustworthy

PATTERNS SMASHED: Co-dependency and people pleasing, shame, the inner critic, over-apologizing, not saying no

WATCHWORD: Kindness

SOUNDTRACK: 'The One and Only' by Chesney Hawkes

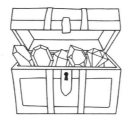

Loving Ourselves

My Greatest Achievement

If you asked me, 'Miranda, what would you say is your greatest achievement?' I'd say, 'Thank you very much for asking such an intriguing question,' and pause thoughtfully and dramatically – perhaps putting my hand on my chin and looking upwards like a real 'thinker'. Although it's an easy answer, I'd do the pause for dramatic effect and to make me look, you know, very profound and things.

The answer is this: my greatest achievement is learning to be kind and compassionate to myself and rewiring my mind away from negative self-talk and judgement. Put another way – less palatable, and easily misconstrued, but I shall say it anyway – my greatest achievement has been falling in love with myself. (MDRC, apologies if that's so cringey to you that you're sinking into your chair. You may want to shake it out or hide behind a cushion for a moment . . .)

I would also include within that potentially icky statement: understanding the science behind self-care, understanding boundaries and how utterly vital they are, learning to say no, saying goodbye to any kind of people-pleasing, and getting to grips with my newly accepted vulnerability – including the 'asking for help' ghastliness. Without a shadow of doubt, these achievements have wholly and profoundly changed my life.

In the past I'd have squirmed at these notions. I wanted to be a strong, powerful, creative, energetic, productive woman and nothing else. Now I know that living strong is not possible without vulnerability. But I suspect that even ten years ago, I would have said my greatest achievement was my sitcom, *Miranda*. It does come a close second for sure.

I was writing a sitcom character whose sole mission was to fall in love with herself. It was a story of how long it takes most women (and I'm sure many men) to stop fitting in and instead love – and be – themselves. I can remember being confused when a female journalist called the show misogynistic. My *Miranda* character was wearing her heart on her sleeve, sharing how difficult it was to be herself in a world that told her she didn't really match up or have a place. I couldn't understand why another woman didn't either identify with that idea or at least agree with how terrible it is that we should ever be made to feel 'wrong' for how we look or feel or who we are. I concluded that she must have been one of the lucky ones – that she must have always felt good about her looks and her general everything-ness. But is there anyone like that, truly?! I'm sounding bitter now, which I'm assuredly not because it was actually a very helpful reaction. It helped me confirm, when writing the show's finale, that I was going to get my character together with the man she'd always loved – but not until she didn't need him to justify herself. She was full of enough worth without a handsome, easy-going man by her side to prove it. Aren't we all? She had to love herself to be free and well (and indeed to love well). Don't we all?

Epiphany

When the truth behind loving oneself slowly settled from my head to my heart, I had an epiphany. The difficult discoveries in the early, dark part of the cave were all pointing to this. This was the treasure of all treasures. The one on which they would all hang. Without self-compassion and kindness, how could I let myself do the things I needed to do to recover? Without kindly accepting my situation how could I share and ask for help? Without lovingly allowing myself to feel and grieve how could I move my story on? Without self-love, how do we start to 'just be ourselves'? Without self-respect and worth, to know we belong, how do we stop people-pleasing and putting on a mask to fit in? Without knowing and loving ourselves, how do we understand what negative thoughts to rewire away from and follow our unique path? Without all of this, might I too end up regretting not living true to myself?

As you know, I have been finding foundational watchwords for each treasure. If this treasure can be tied up in one word, it's this: kindness. Kindness is what we all need. It's another aspect of our inherent identity. I truly believe that accepting, respecting and being kind to ourselves can be the greatest life-changer. Remember, there is a point in you and your life! We *all* matter. Richard Rohr, a Franciscan friar, puts it majestically:

So many of us carry a kind of unspoken assumption that something is very, very wrong with us, that we're damaged,

guilty and unlovable ... acknowledging and accepting our
fundamental nobility is the ultimate paradigm shift.

Wow. MDRC, now I've declared this epiphany, I shall share how it all came about. Particularly as this treasure culminated in an extraordinary heavy revvy – the heaviest of revelations for me. What a tease ...

Science Of Self-Care

It started when I came across a social media post of a woman extolling the virtues of self-care. She was lying on a soft, luscious rug in a Norwegian log cabin with a rugged, bearded, kind-eyed man passing her a hot chocolate. I remember thinking, *Umm, hang on, that's not self-care – that's a privileged mini-break, isn't it?* If we're led to believe that self-care means having the money, health and luck to have a gorgeous, gentle Viking of a man chop wood for our log fire as we pose, laughing, our long blonde locks brushing a tiny marshmallow off the top of a foaming hot chocolate, we're assuredly on very rocky ground! It's yet more propaganda to make us feel we're lacking. And it perpetuates the lie that if we're crippled by illness or poverty or burn-out or isolation, then self-compassion and -esteem isn't something we can find. I started the journey to self-compassion with the tiniest acts from the confinement of a bed. In your face, Norwegian chalet breaks! (Though obviously they look amazing. Just not as a solution for self-care.)

It seems to me we are in a grey area with this self-care malarkey. People might say, 'Have a self-care weekend,' or, 'Don't forget to look after yourself.' Self-care is a hashtag. We bandy it about. And that's okay, and better than not being aware of it at all. But it's too important a thing just to bandy. If someone who is struggling believes that self-care is just a treat, like a bubble bath with a take-away pizza – if they haven't been taught what self-care is practically, physiologically and emotionally – then after a bath and a shot of carbs they will feel a bit hotter and on a brief sugar high before the cold, baseline discontent returns. We try to be kind to ourselves, nothing changes, so we go back to familiar ways which then allow unhelpful patterns to continue. We need to understand the science behind self-care.

I was frustrated that it wasn't intrinsically in me to nurture self-compassion. Another thing I wish had been on the school syllabus. Here I was, a reasonably clever (say nothing) middle-aged woman, suddenly facing the fact that there had been a bizarre and unknowingly small amount of self-compassion in her life. I had never been taught its relevance and vitality – how humbling, how infuriating. I had no choice but to learn a tiny bit more of the science.

Right, we can do this, MDRC. I will guide you towards my heaviest revvy as simply as I can. The first bit of study makes me sound vaguely academic for a brief momento, but don't worry. I'll fart soon and tell you what it sounds like and all will be back to normal. For now, please do concentrate!

So, get this: it can sometimes be hard to foster self-compassion because we all have an ingrained, natural 'negativity bias'. We've evolved to focus on our mistakes more than our successes, so we can right any wrongs to keep us connected for survival. Clever, eh? Because we're wired to belong, we're naturally concerned about our reputation and want to be respected within our community.

Our first 'community', our first connection, is with our family. The safety of feeling known and understood, of being 'seen', is what allows us to develop a healthy brain and nervous system while gaining a sense of self. As children, we need to know our needs are going to be met, because that is what eventually teaches us to meet our own needs, developing self-protection, expression and esteem. But, as you will remember, not every child will get that sense of safe connection. The inner critic can then develop.

And, so, get this. If we start to repeatedly accredit negative value to ourselves when it's not necessary, criticism becomes harmful. (That, incidentally, is why we have a conscience – we always know when we have gone truly wrong and need to apologize.) I am sure most of us at one time in our lives have hit the pillow after a social event and had racing thoughts that we are idiots who have committed some kind of serious social offence just by spitting sausage roll pastry on to someone's face – just me? *Any* criticism is perceived as a threat to the brain and body. This means that self-criticism can put us on a high-alert fear response. Get this quote from Dr Richard Davidson, known for his groundbreaking work on emotion and the brain:

> *Self-criticism can take a toll on our minds and bodies. It can lead to ruminative thoughts that interfere with our productivity, and it can impact our bodies by stimulating inflammatory mechanisms that lead to chronic illness and accelerate aging.*

I'm not glad that it was a long-term illness that introduced me to the effects of the inner critic (aka a lack of self-compassion), but I'm glad I got to meet her so that I could free myself from her. And with that, MDRC, here was my personal revelation of revelations in the middle of my unexpected decade of darkness and within the middle of my metaphorical cave. It's specifically about the situation I was in, but I really hope that it could be life-changing for you too.

Bear with, as I try and explain it as best I can. Okay, here goes. Imagine the nervous system works within a pot (or a jug – whatever receptacle works for you!). A stress pot. A pot that ranges from relaxed at 1 to total overwhelm at 10. If we feel nice and calm and life feels possible and manageable, our nervous system might be functioning with a task at a 2 or 3 out of 10. The stress pot has lots of room – if there is a difficult situation to deal with, like an emergency at work or a health issue in the family or a car breakdown mid-journey, the nervous system will respond with stress. This fear response fires up the limbic survival part of the brain to get the heart racing, the blood going to the muscles and the tunnel vision for the necessary singular focus to deal with the threat. It might take you to a stress level of 7 or 8 out of 10 to deal with the situation, but your stress pot will slowly come back down when the danger is over. This is a nervous system working well. MDRC, forgive me if you already know these things, but what I've described above is the nervous system naturally going into a flight-or-fight response. Sometimes it might go into a freeze state of shutdown (when the best defence against a threat might have been, historically, to 'play dead' and get into the foetal position – and indeed something that might be right for us to do now at times). We are meant to experience stress. The nervous system is designed to go up and down throughout the day for various reasons – one example being performance anxiety, which can give us energy for a particular task.

The thing that I didn't know – my life-changing revvy – was that our stress pots can get stuck on full. We may then perpetually operate at a 9 out of 10 without respite, which in time leads to a chronic stress response. Unlike a normal anxiety response that goes up and down, chronic stress means one's system is in a permanent state of high alert All The Time. Getting stuck in this state can cause complications – symptoms like, unsurprisingly, exhaustion, not waking up refreshed, irritability, a feeling of being overwhelmed, sleeplessness, muscle tension, migraine, fatigue, discontent. Not such fun, but I wouldn't be sharing if I hadn't discovered there are ways to heal, ways to bring our stress pots back down to manageable levels. Dig in with me if you so desire . . .

Basically, with chronic stress our physical and emotional selves can't function properly. The brain thinks we are always under threat, so it doesn't have time for joy and play and optimism. If this state goes on for long enough, we can end up with secondary issues like pain, arthritis, skin problems, food sensitivities or IBS. Stick with me if you are relating to any of this because there's light at the end of the cave. I promise.

We might end up in a chronic stress state for a number of reasons – a combination of lack of good sleep and food while overworking, causing burn-out, is common nowadays. It could be from PTSD, or complex childhood trauma. It's usually a slow accumulation of stressors over many years that tips us into chronic stress, which is why it's often hard to see what's happened. That's what had happened to me.

The physical stress of viral infections and injuries was my primary stressor (the body comes under huge stress when fighting disease ...). The years of fear from misdiagnosis added to my stress pot. Physical conditions like hypermobility and PoTS added. My workload added (even though I loved it and wanted it). The simple fact of living in a busy city in a frantic world added. All the bad patterns I had got into added. Then, of course, there was the stress of stress. Thoughts like, *Will I get through the day?*, *Should I eat this or will it cause a migraine?*, *Am I doing too much or not enough?* (I'm pretty sure whatever our trickiest life thing is, MDRC, we have looping thoughts about it – and in my experience that can often become the worst problem.)

I also saw that a lack of self-compassion, self-respect, self-love – and the resultant toxicity from negative thoughts or bad habits – would of course be contributing. For years, I had been waking up with symptoms that I now see were being caused by a stress pot at a 9 out of 10, due to my undiagnosed Lyme and associated infections from immune system disorder. Anything I then had to do that day would cause extreme fatigue. That's why I eventually collapsed.

I don't want to leap ahead because I have a final part of this heavy revelation to share – but, to keep you going, MDRC, I now call it an exciting revelation, because if I could slowly remove stress from my pot, then my body could get back to some efficient functioning to recover. *Keep calm, Miranda, carry on finishing the science ...*

Get this. Have you noticed how you can feel low and fatigued and even anxious when you have a cold or flu? Well, that's because the immune system correctly fires up to get rid of the invader. The immune system is linked to the nervous system, and that heightens too. The immune system, after receiving the message from our brain, cleverly gives us symptoms to put us to bed while making sure we do what we need to do for the infection to leave. It's not the disease causing the symptoms, it's our brain. MIND-BLOWING. Cue symptoms of anxiety or a feeling of being wired or difficulty sleeping mixed with groggy fatigue. When the cold virus is cleared out, the brain gets off its fight, flight or freeze alert response – the threat has gone. Our body is doing exactly what it's designed to do.

There's more! If we already have a full stress pot by order of current life circumstances, the immune system isn't going to work efficiently. If we catch a virus or infection when our immune system is dysregulated in this way, it can't clear it. It is already working overtime and so it shouts, 'Help, we don't have enough resources to clear this infection – throw more at it.' The nervous and immune systems then fire up further, causing inflammation and even more gross symptoms than normal.

And, so, drumroll, GET THIS – evidence now suggests that *this* is how long-term conditions such as long Covid and ME/chronic fatigue syndrome (CFS) start. Basically, when the acute virus has left the body, the immune system Never Gets The Message. It continues to pour adrenalin into the body to fight the disease. The fatigue persists, other latent viruses reactivate and secondary problems and symptoms occur because the brain is still on high alert. That's the condition in a nutshell. ME was called 'yuppie flu' when it started being registered more and more in the eighties. This makes sense to me now. High-functioning, highly wired, fast-paced city workers and the like were getting it because their stress pots were at a 10 out of 10 just by living. (Of course, something not exclusive to city workers.) One virus would be enough to cause the condition, as the body couldn't function to clear it. Many people that I know who have had CFS or long Covid or chronic pain say that before they got sick, they were in a period of stress and/or difficulty. Lots of university students burning the candle at both ends, lots of athletes pushing their bodies to the limit, lots of mothers working long hours. For others, it's that unknowing build-up of stress – which is why I am so passionate about smashing unserving worldly patterns, because it was becoming clear they perpetuate stress.

Yup, there it was – it wouldn't be until my stress response reduced that my nervous system and immune system could go back to any kind of homeostasis. Until this happened, my body wouldn't be able to clear the Lyme and other infections ravaging me. I finally understood why getting out of bed eventually became a no-go for my dear body.

It's so very important to make it clear that this is a physical condition. For thirty-five years I was told I had anxiety as my body got sicker and sicker – but ME/CFS, long Covid and others are not anxiety conditions (or cries for help or laziness, as people can still be absurdly labelled). There is immune system disorder, autoimmune issues, there is viral load, energy cells might be severely depleted, and so on (some people end up on oxygen). But the cause and the solution are in the brain's heightened stress response.

So, join my excitement despite it all if you can, MDRC. This was the greatest revelation because I now know that my brain is plastic. I can work with my mind to tell my brain that the threat is over, thereby helping my immune system to finally function as it is meant to. EXTRAORDINARY.

Suddenly, all the treasures were shining beacons that made sense in a scientific, diagnostic way – reduce stress, meet your needs, look after yourself, take pressure off yourself to constantly 'be better'. Love yourself. Not because it's a nice-sounding idea but because it leads to good health. I felt like I finally had some kind of manual. I had ways to put myself back in the world in an authentic and calm way, to function well instead of trying to fit in with the world's pace.

As Dr Kristin Neff, self-compassion expert extraordinaire, says in her book *Self-Compassion* (good title), 'Our culture does not emphasize self-compassion, quite the opposite. We're told that no matter how hard we try, our best just isn't good enough.' We have to learn to soothe ourselves. Or, as the 'ists' say, to 'reparent ourselves'. Certainly, this made sense with what I continued to learn in this treasure.

If the science of self-care is ultimately about meeting our vital needs to reduce an overwhelmed stress pot, then when we *intentionally* have a bubble bath and a take-away pizza because, for example, we have said no to something we knew we didn't have capacity for – and so stopped ourselves from people-pleasing to prove we are loved – we are rewiring old patterns. The act changes us, thereby becoming true self-care.

Well, that was a lot of information, MDRC. I need to take a breather. Even writing about it again, I need to savour the relief of knowing it. Shall we have a lie-down? (Not together – steady . . .) But I hope you're excited or at least hopeful or intrigued. Our discontent – however it is manifesting, perhaps longing to just feel less tired – really can shift. Onwards!

P.S. As promised – I just farted, and it sounded like a creaky haunted house door. You're welcome . . .

The Beautiful Bluebell Bulb

Even with delving into and accepting the clear science (and hearing of thousands of people cured from similar conditions to mine), there was still a part of me from the past that would occasionally pop up and question whether 'loving yourself' really was the ultimate answer, and the place to start. It's easy to think the small actions towards that each day are trite or can't really be making physical change. My attention was grabbed and understanding firmly pinned down in an intriguing way. It was via a lovely wooden crate of bluebell bulbs.

I'd been stuck inside again with a flare-up of viral symptoms (shingles this time – hello to those lovely 'temporary tattoos'!), and a friend kindly brought some nature to brighten up my literal and metaphorical insides. The bulbs were sitting quite high in the soil and a few green shoots had begun emerging from each. I could already imagine their beauty in full bloom and easily visualized the wooded carpet that I longed to walk in. It was unlikely I would get to the wood for real that year, so I decided to love those little bulbs and watch them grow.

I was reminded of an experiment that had been done on plants in a children's classroom. The teacher had heard about the fascinating 'rice experiment' – a professor, Dr Masaru Emoto, put two bowls of the same cooked rice in a fridge; he spoke loving words over one bowl and vile, toxic words over the other. The bowl spoken badly over started going mouldy in a way the other didn't. I KNOW! Talk about the power of words. The teacher gave the schoolkids plants to look after for their version of the experiment. They spoke loving words over some of the plants and noticed they grew, while the ones they spoke horrible words over withered. Extraordinary and shocking. For there it was in plain sight – the reality of the energetic matter of negative thoughts and what criticism can do to us. And the necessity of kindness.

I decided to do my own experiment. I looked at my beautiful bluebell bulbs, chose one in the corner, touched it and started speaking similar words that I had heard my inner critic shout about my illness that day. Things like 'it's your fault', 'you let yourself down yesterday', 'you're never going to get well'. An unexpected thing happened – projecting those words on to an innocent living thing was more heart-rendingly painful than I could have imagined. I could hardly keep going; it felt wrong to be so cruel even to a bluebell bulb.

If it pains us to hurt another, it also pains us to hurt ourselves. In that moment I knew I could never entertain my inner critic again. Let alone when this happened: the bulb that I touched every day for a week, the one I disparaged with words like 'you will never bloom', 'you are not as good as the rest of these bulbs' . . . well, it barely grew. It was at *least* half the size of the others. The others were tall, proud, strong and surrounded by three or four smaller offshoots. The one I'd been mean to was shorter with not a single offshoot. Watching this happen before my eyes – and not just on paper as a research study – forever changed me.

I was also struck – and this undid me – by how easy it had become, after that guilt-inducing first day, to 'abuse' that bluebell bulb. I had quickly become desensitized. I guessed that this was because, subconsciously, I was used to directing these unkind thoughts at myself. From here on out, I was going to do all I could to fuel my life with self-compassion and kindness.

We are not what our inner critics say we are.

Pipe Down, Sandy!

Before we journey onwards, here's an amusing but genius way to dismantle an inner critic that may be affecting you that I discovered from Martha Beck, Kristin Neff and Steven Hayes (all the 'ists' would agree). They suggest naming and picturing one's inner critic (we all have one but to varying degrees). This might sound like more, rather than less, madness, but I found it such a powerful act. If, as you dare to get to know your top ten thought tunes, and a character of the critic forms, my advice is to lean into it. Our critics will all be different.

Without further ado I would like to introduce you to mine: Sergeant Major Sandy! She wears a safari outfit – wide khaki shorts to the knees and long white socks pulled up. And a hard hat – obviously. She's the one who gets stressed when we are late, wants everything done *immediately*, hates anything left on a to-do list, doesn't want to waste a single moment. And I don't actually mind that about her. People who know me well can see when I'm siding with Sandy . . . and they like it because a holiday gets booked, things get done and tidied, a comedy show gets drilled so hard in rehearsals we make it look and feel effortless in front of an audience (if I may be so bold). Sandy will be checking Google Maps to make sure we don't sit in traffic unnecessarily (always leaving an extra half an hour early anyway), would never miss a plane and always has an emergency energy bar in her bag. We all need a Sandy to a certain extent (each of us has that planning and organizing part of our brain). The problem is when she tips into sergeant major mode and paces about, puts her hard hat on and gets out a whip! Then she tells me I am lazy and that I should be getting up at five in the morning like she has heard those people on Instagram say is the way to max the day. She thinks I am ridiculous when I tell her my body clock suits getting up at eight or nine if I can. She berates any lack of physical fitness and muscle tone, leaving no space for me to explain that it isn't my fault of late. And she used to not like my face. RUDE! She plans ahead constantly and doesn't see the point of sitting still in the present. She can't be bothered with emotion, she just wants to crack on and do. And she'll tell me at the end of every day what I could have done better.

Naming and picturing her really did work. I could laugh at her. I could celebrate what I liked about her, and then I could start to say, 'Oh, do pipe down, Sandy,' when it was an attack that didn't serve me, or I knew would put stress on my body.

I was in charge because I had brought her out of the subconscious. It wasn't madness but genius from the 'ists'. It was the ultimate kindness.

Doing this work is profound. It's like setting yourself free from prison. I knew the revelatory diagnosis that my body was in a chronic stress response was right, for whenever I told Sandy to pipe down, I felt a change in my body. Similarly, when I surrendered and felt or expressed emotion, there was a release of tension. My stress pot was being reduced.

At the core, it was self-compassion.

Don't Go Breaking My Heart

I did wonder whether this central treasure on loving ourselves was preparing me for a romantic relationship. I was thinking of The Boy from Bristol more and more. We were FaceTiming quite a bit between sofa-chatting days. One evening, he told me I looked beautiful. My past response would have been something akin to, 'Oh now, stop it, well, I'm a mess, okay, to you maybe, but you just probably don't have your glasses on, I don't know . . . [pulls weird face and giggles].' This time, I put my learnings into practice. I said . . . 'Thank you.' It felt surprisingly alien, but strong, and 'right'. Not just because I FaceTimed with the camera in a flattering low light. One step at a time!

Whether I was preparing myself for a relationship or not, I knew I had to just let it unfold (hark at me surrendering). I was following in the footsteps of my penned sitcom

199

character, not *needing* another to complete me but *wanting* another to love and be loved by. The journey into self-compassion is knowing we are enough on our own. We cannot get our worth from outside of ourselves. I had taken both those truths to heart, and I was not going to fall into the trap of idealizing a romantic partner as a saviour. No, siree!

My thinking developed further (I fancied myself quite the philosopher by now). MDRC, I wondered: can you really love, truly, if you're wearing a mask of any kind? Surely sincere love means the ability to show the truth of who we are, reveal and be revealed without shame or judgement? If I loved myself, I could freely drop the masks and instead be honest about who I was. Which meant that I could be loved and love better. That continued to be my mission, whether The Boy from Bristol would end up being my person or a person put in my way to learn from.

The next time we FaceTimed I was given another chance to be honestly me. We were about to finish the call when he asked what I was doing with the rest of my evening. I replied, 'I'm going to do some Lego.' A slight pause. He said, 'Sorry, did you say you were going to play Lego?!' I ploughed confidently on. 'Yes, I did. I'm building the Lego Boutique Hotel for the village I'm slowly collecting.' If you are worried that was too much, MDRC, then you might squirm when I say I moved the camera to show him my build (not a euphemism) and introduced him to Dave and Valerie, the Lego people hotel owners. 'Do they come with names?' he asked. 'No,' I said, continuing in all my sexy glory, 'I name them myself.' As I hit the pillow that night, I had to tell Sandy to very much pipe down!

In her book *The Way of Integrity*, Martha Beck cites a study which found that when people told just three fewer white lies a week (like saying no when they might have said yes to ingratiate), they reduced negative emotions and had fewer health problems. I find that COMPLETELY FASCINAT-ING. I know it would have my broken heart a little and weakened me if I had lied to The Boy from Bristol. Everything was telling me to keep on course to free my wild, true self.

Have we aligned too much with the inner critic or outer worldly ways that we have forgotten who we are? There is a quote attributed to Indian philosopher Jiddu Krishnamurti that I had to take a breath on reading: 'It is no measure of health to be well-adjusted to a profoundly sick society.' Wow, perhaps the world's ways are our greatest stressor, I pon-dered ever more philosophically. Perhaps not loving ourselves or looking after ourselves well by the very act of trying to keep up with the world is, in itself, enough to tip the nervous and immune systems into chronic stress.

It was time to delve into patterns that made loving myself so hard, or not naturally part of my life. Uncovering any dam-aging or unhelpful patterns would reveal the practical ways to love myself, not to mention the hope I had for the physiologi-cal shift this could cause. I was revved up on my heavy revvy . . .

Dance Break

A dance break now, Miranda, I hear you say? I know, you're chomping at the bit to gallop towards loving myself by dismantling some hindering habits. Oh, I do love your enthusiasm, MDRC. But what better way to start than by popping on Chesney Hawkes and having a bop (if you are able) to 'The One and Only'.

And some of the patterns are quite, what I call, full on! I hope to serve as the seed sower here, and wish you all the love and the luck in the world if you need to delve into areas that resonate. It will be worth it to reduce your stress pot and release the glorious, wild, true you. You are, MDRC, the one and only . . .

Isn't It Selfish?

Even with academics and researchers telling us that loving ourselves is the way to love better and be healthy, we often *still* think it's selfish (bless us, but also, can we just stop it?!). Self-care cannot be a selfish act. It's scientifically and spiritually impossible. One aspect of human rights is treating each person with respect and dignity and of infinite value. You could therefore say that when we don't treat ourselves accordingly, we are in violation of our own basic human rights. As the Buddhist traditions say, universal human compassion that does not include the self is not universal. Accepting this was a huge relief to me during my fallow time. Much like being told to put our oxygen masks on first before helping another on a plane, I had to dwell on myself for a moment so that I could think of myself less in the end.

The plain fact is that the most loving people love themselves. They know how to love well. That's the paradox here. We don't love ourselves to feel better than another, but as part of being able to show more love and kindness to the heartbreak of this world. If we love ourselves, we look after ourselves. And the healthier we are, the more energy we have for our families, work and acts of kindness. Conversely, when we try and be something we aren't to please others, it's exhausting and untrue, leaving less space to look and serve outwards.

Self-care is not selfish; it could in fact change the world! Parker J. Palmer in his wonderful short book *Let Your Life Speak* sums it up perfectly:

> *Self-care is never a selfish act – it is simply good stewardship of the only gift I have, the gift I was put on earth to offer others. Anytime we can listen to true self and give the care it requires, we do it not only for ourselves but for the many others whose lives we touch.*

Boom – he nailed it!

Plus, I often just think: I'm lumbered with me – I'd rather love me than not!

'Tut-Tut – Sorry, Sorry'

Still, now, when I spill something or get something wrong, I might automatically say out loud, 'Oh, Miranda,' in a ticking-off way. Not a massively big deal but it all adds up. I immediately now replace this with, 'Pipe down, Sandy, I'm still loved, every-body makes mistakes,' to make sure these little 'attacks' don't add to my stress pot. It's not on my side to 'tut' myself! Not what a faithful friend or kind parent would do. (By the way, all the 'ists' say that a simple route to start loving yourself is to check whether what you are thinking or doing is what you would kindly do for a friend in the same position.)

And how many times do we say the S-word, MDRC? Sorry.

Sorry, my hair's a mess.

Sorry, I'm a bit emotional today.

Sorry, I look really scruffy.

Sorry I didn't get back to you sooner (after half an hour without replying to an email).

Sorry, am I early? Oh sorry, I don't like to be the first, are you ready for me?

Sorry, am I late? So sorry, I hate being the last, hope I haven't caused a prob.

Sorry, I misheard you, sorry, I don't know what's wrong with me today. I must be overtired, sorry.

Someone knocks into us in the street – 'I'm so sorry.'

Someone lets us go first in a shop doorway – 'Sorry.'

Sorry I exist, really. Just one big fat soz to the world.

STOP IT!

My route to stopping my tut-ing and my sorry-ing was via the power of channelling Beyoncé at a zebra crossing! I had made a vow to myself not to say sorry again unless I needed to, but when, a few days after making said vow, I walked across a zebra crossing, I noticed my typical hand up to thank the car for stopping, my head bowed and my lowly stance as I rushed across. *Hang on*, I thought, *it's their duty to stop. Next time, I am not going to be remotely apologetic.* And when that day came, I waited at the pavement, the cars stopped, and I put my shoulders back and pranced majestically Beyoncé-style for all womankind who have been conditioned to apologize when they don't need to. It felt amazing. I hasten to add that I am not condoning obnoxious behaviour. I actually found by not scraping and bowing in apology for crossing a road meant I felt a better version of myself and had the energy to smile heartily at the cars. It was an added bonus that I felt powerful and sexy and wish someone had been on the other side with a wind machine for full effect!

Oh God, I Have Needs!

Since Treasure One, what had been brewing and bubbling to the surface was that there would be no avoiding getting to know my own needs. But, if you're like me, you might not *like* the idea of having needs. With the world having told me that it was stronger to be fierce and independent, the idea of needing needs still aggravated. I did not want to need needs. I was feeling all the nuance of the human condition around this. I knew it was scary for my nervous system to crack on and not have my needs met, and that made me feel like a shaky little dormouse. I also knew it was important to claim what I needed to take the right action to look after myself. Yes, that felt good; I sat up stronger, more like a plump guinea pig (I think we all know I should desist on the animal metaphors.). Then I thought, hang on, nope, needs are officially shit – they sometimes mean you have to ask for help. But . . . I knew I couldn't love and look after myself if I didn't accept my vulnerability at times. I was going to go for it, MDRC. I was going to master asking for help.

The first time I asked for help in Treasure One, I was cowering behind a door frame. This next attempt I went the other way. Strident. I went popstar again, shoulders back, tits out, and strode purposefully round to my neighbour's to ask a favour. It went something a bit like this:

'Hi there, sorry to disturb. I mean, no, I'm not sorry. Sorry. Let me start again.'

Takes deep breath, realizes the tits out thing is a bit weird so casually places hand on hip.

'Right, so here's the thing . . . Question . . .' *Starts singing 'Independent Women'.*

Realizes have made myself laugh singing Beyoncé and quickly desist.

Neighbour: 'Were you just singing Destiny's Child?'

'Yes, but that's fine, yup, sorry, not sorry, no it's . . . I do have a question . . .'

Can't help but do a Beyoncé-esque move.

'Right. I've got a question – don't need to tell me what you think about me because I'm fabulous . . . Ignore me . . . Except, I wondered . . . Question: I don't suppose you could do me a huge favour and take my dog to the vet around the corner this afternoon? I'm still shielding and it's quite a small space.'

Puts hand over mouth to prevent saying, 'No probs if not.'

Neighbour: 'Yes, of course, I'm working from home, it will be a nice break.'

'Right, okay, oh, wow, that was easy . . . great, thank you. Is that that, then? Great, lovely, thanks.'

End scene.

Yes, I went a bit weird. Beyoncé on a day off. But I did it! And they were kind. It would have been fine if they'd said no, too, but by asking each other for help we give each other the chance to feel good about helping. Humans are inherently kind; we like to help.

(It's a shame that my neighbour's visit coincided with the vet saying my dear doggy needed to have her anal glands unblocked. She might not have said yes if she knew she was going to face the sight (gross) and smell (fishy) of that, but in my defence I didn't know that was going to happen . . . Moving on . . .)

Pleasing The Peoples Or Codependency –
Now What?!

There I was, still reeling from needing needs, when I was next faced with the idea of codependency. Expert 'ist' in this area Pia Mellody defines codependency as the chronic neglect of self to gain approval, love or validation through another person. Ouch, heartbreaking.

It can manifest in fear of upsetting anyone, always being the carer, low self-worth, remaining in tricky relationships out of guilt, taking on the advisor role and constantly fixing others, finding it hard to communicate one's own ideas and wants. All the opposite of loving oneself. And most of which I felt extremely blessed not to live under.

MDRC, it's such a colossal waste of time, protecting ourselves by looking out for what people might think about us. We can never know what people will think of us. As I recently heard Mel Robbins say on her podcast, 'You will never, ever live a life you are meant to live if you are constantly worried what other people are thinking. Two things can be true at the same time – people can have opinions about you and still love you.'

So, for example, shall we try and stop doing the, 'What do you want, whatever you want, I don't mind, well you go first, no after you . . .' It's EXHAUSTING! People-pleasing says you shouldn't state your needs, you should follow the pack. But, as I say, clarity is kindness and we need to keep freeing ourselves, stating our likes and dislikes. (P.S. On which note, The Boy liked my Lego! I'm digressing, but for good reason, as you will see . . .).

I get mildly irritated when I say, 'Shall we eat?' and the reply is, 'I don't mind, maybe, I could eat.' And I think, *Well, I know you could eat. I've seen you, you're very good at the eating, you can use a knife and fork and everything. I know you could eat, but do you want to or not?* It's so utterly lovely if someone gleefully says, 'I would really love to eat,' or decisively says, 'Thanks, but I'm not hungry.' We have an infinitely better time.

If I am sounding rather smug because I don't suffer from this often at times very debilitating trait, don't worry, I was firmly put in my place. I read in Pia Mellody's book *Codependency* (another woman good at titles) that it is *also* neglecting of the self to be anti-dependent, invulnerable, controlling (though I like to say wise!), capable, hard- or overworking. Which is why codependency isn't spotted in many independent and 'successful' people. NOW WHAT?! So I have been codependent? RUDE!

But I am grateful, as her theory cemented for me, once and for all, that such traits, despite still often lauded, are clearly not kind or loving to oneself, and would contribute heavily to the stress pot. Luckily, with Treasure One firmly in my pocket, I was slowly walking out of those ways.

What Are Boundaries? And Now What?!

Another word bandied about is 'boundaries'. But how many of us *really* know what it means? I didn't. More studying for me.

Boundaries are our clear lines and limits. The ways we protect ourselves from others, physically and emotionally. Without them it's hard to love and protect ourselves and easily leads to reduced energy. A boundary could be how close we let another person come to us or being clear and firm with our sister for reading our diary. When we have strong and healthy boundaries, we take responsibility for our thinking, feelings and behaviour and keep them separate from others'. We don't blame anyone else for what we think, feel and do (yes, mull on that one), nor do we take responsibility for the actions of others. Just the thought of that and I relax a little.

Boundaries lead to healthier ways to live, such as taking care of ourselves, respecting ourselves so that we are treated as equals, feeling safe to express emotions, being okay with disagreements, and knowing who we are and what we like.

It all sounded good in theory.

But hang on un petit momento (a sexy little French–Italian combo there . . .) – here was all the nuance again, all the ins and outs of humanness. To move into self-love I had to accept a degree of vulnerability and ask for help, likely making me a babbling, tearful mess at times. But I also had to be firm in stating my precise and exact boundaries and, head held high, say what I needed – nay, demanded! To someone I know. And at the risk of them not understanding or being cross with me or thinking I was rude. EVEN THE NOTION! On top of that, the 'ists' told me that being misunderstood was going to be part of the process. FOR GOODNESS' SAKE – NOW WHAT?!

It helped me understand the nuance of boundaries all the more when I saw how amusingly scary it was to first start setting them. Being housebound was not the easiest way but opportunities did arise. This was the first one . . .

A friend had popped in for a cup of tea and on realizing she was late for a meeting, she rushed out and quickly asked me, 'Do you mind if I pop in on the way back and use your printer?'

She was, of course, expecting a simple yes. And in the past it would have been. Because that's what you 'should' do.

But by then I was more intentional, and in this instance I knew I was very tired and part of recovery at the time was needing the evening undisturbed. (Obviously if she was having any kind of emergency, I would have considered how I might be capable of helping.) I went for it, MDRC.

I said, 'No, actually, that doesn't work for me this evening.'

There was a pause.

She looked at me as if I'd said, 'Do you mind if I just do a poo in your mouth?' (Sorry!)

The pause continued but the new boundaried me was determined not to back down. I couldn't not fill the gap so I explained, 'I know it's hard to understand but I really need a quiet night to myself . . .'

She stared again, as if I had asked her to throw a small kitten into a river. (Sorry!)

And then she said, 'No, of course, nice idea, I can probably ask my husband anyway. Wow, gosh, have a lovely evening. Wow, that's so brilliant of you. Amazing.' She was acting as if I'd just won the Nobel Peace Prize. I could see it had made her think – are we really allowed to say what we need?

Yes, we are! And it was absolutely another key way I started to regain energy and feel more honestly me. A lack of boundaries can significantly add to the stress pot.

It was a relief to learn that having limits with others, to protect ourselves and our energy, doesn't mean you don't love them. In fact, the opposite. People in good and safe relationships respect each other's empowering and resourcing boundaries. It can be the secret to loving more.

Saying No – Now What, Please?!

Right, so if we're going to have boundaries, we're going to have to say no. I know – NOW WHAT?!

Just say no. Respect yourself. Don't under-resource yourself. It should be easy. It's not, though, is it, MDRC? It means undoing a whole lot more worldly conditioning. And it takes time. For what it's worth, I can't begin to explain how valuable it was for me.

To my mind, the honesty of a 'no' can't be rivalled. It's reminiscent of honourably gathering or not gathering at all. With a 'no' firmly in our vocabulary, our yeses will mean so much more (they will never be people-pleasing white lies) and we will be acting kindly and resourcefully. I love people who say no. I always feel free to ask them for help. I trust them. I know when they say yes, they want to be there wholeheartedly. It's so loving. It's true kindness. Clarity is kindness!

When I Cancelled Christmas!

It turns out if you can say no to Christmas, you can say no to anything. I was meant to be going to my parents' house for Christmas. A natural, time-honoured tradition. That's what we do at Christmas, isn't it? We go home, we have a duty to our family. Or, rather, we want to be with them, to celebrate them, to give them gifts, to be light and love for the light and love season. But then sometimes, we just don't. Christmas for me is never normally a weighty duty. I love spending it with my family. Except this particular year, I just did not want to. I was feeling particularly unwell. I'd recently come back from an overnight trip (something still quite new to me energy-wise) and my body was yearning to stay in my own home, not pack again, be in my own bed, and have some quiet, hunkering winter time. But I couldn't cancel Christmas, could I? Of course I couldn't, it would be mean and wrong . . . I spent the next few days trying to rest so that I would feel up to going (this felt familiar), but I just kept getting more stressed and upset. Why? Because I wasn't doing what I needed to do. It came to 23 December and I knew I had to cancel. I felt I was doing the most terrifyingly rude, selfish act a human could do. Who was I fearing admonishment from? I have no idea. Would I still love myself, and did I know this was the right decision? Yes.

In the end, all that happened was that my mother was incredibly understanding. She didn't want me to be under any pressure, it was all okay.

I got off the call and, yup, it happened again. Proof. My body relaxed, some fatigue lifted. I felt a pressure literally come off me. I spent Christmas alone. That didn't matter. It was just any other day to me that year. It turned out I had shingles again, which was why I was feeling so bad. I had made the right call.

It was an amazing (self-)gift to have had the chance to cancel Christmas. Who cancels Christmas?! But it was as if my soul was saying, 'Finally. Thank you.' We never let ourselves down when we listen to and respect our needs and boundaries, when we let go of past patterns or say no. Never. We let ourselves up.

The Taxi Driver

When my health improved enough that I could actually be in the world and interact with other humans again, I had more chances to put boundaries in place. I was excited. There's so much of life that I can't control which can cause angst, so I wanted to help myself as best I could by doing things to naturally keep reducing stress and hopefully feel more well. It felt like an exciting threshold, MDRC . . . until I was faced with how absurdly difficult maintaining boundaries is in the real world!

I was in a taxi, and in a fairly common situation that might require a boundary, the lovely driver embarked upon the non-stop chatter. At a time I did not feel I had the energy or desire to engage. And I do mean *non-stop* chat. Barely a breath between sentences. It's strange when people just launch into their life story, isn't it? With no encouragement, they're just off and it's very hard to stop them! All I needed to simply say was, 'I'm tired and need to sit in silence, so I can't chat at the moment, thanks so much.' But that's not what nice, polite people do, is it? And I didn't want to cause a fuss. I couldn't believe how I, a confident and indeed often opinionated middle-aged woman, wasn't able to find those words. Ridiculous! STOP IT!

I thought how easy it would be to return home and moan, 'Blooming taxi driver didn't draw breath – so insensitive, I'm knackered.' And, MDRC, this is when the world of boundary is at its peak power. Because the taxi driver wasn't being remotely insensitive. I hadn't asked him to stop talking. He thought he had a kindly ear. He was doing nothing wrong. Oh, how often we can blame another when it was not their fault, but ours for not saying we needed them to stop talking or whatever their stress-inducing action for us was. How often do we gossip about another's behaviour when we allowed them to behave that way? No one is a mind-reader. Give people a chance. It's a massive twist and game-changer.

215

I sat in the back of the taxi, feeling overwhelmed by his loud voice and overlapping sentences, and started to respond with those supposedly polite but ultimately unloving – nay, seething – 'umms' and 'yeahs' between sentences. Nope, I didn't want to be that person. I took a deep breath, was amused at a slight heart-racing anxiety (my brain perceiving this new way as a danger lest I am not liked), and said, 'Excuse me, could I just have five minutes to myself? Just need to shut my eyes for a moment.' He simply said, 'Yeah, course, you just relax back there,' and was immediately quiet.

I felt relief and smiled at how utterly absurd it was that it had been hard for me to ask for something so simple. And then, knowing I could meet my needs and stop listening at any time, I felt a freedom to listen. I wanted to listen. After ten minutes I said, 'So, what were you saying . . . ?' And he was off! And I am so glad I heard his story.

He was a foster carer, as well as having two children of his own. He was brought up in Bermondsey, South London, but his community had been priced out of the area, and many couldn't feed or house their kids. He'd gathered up as many kids as he and his wife could cope with. He and his wife were letting go of the savings they had put aside for holidays and other hard-earned comforts to help. It was a story of joyful sacrifice. And it inspired me. This man had a self-confidence about him that he was doing the best he could, what he needed to do, and he seemed to be so alive. He had many challenges, but he was following who he was and I just knew he was somebody who could say no if he needed to (other-wise I don't think he would have been able to say yes to what he already had).

He had kindness pouring out of every pore. It reminded me that kindness and love is like a stick of rock going through our DNA when we are functioning at our best, whatever we do, wherever we are from. And he was flourishing because of his.

Perhaps he was resourced in loving himself in all the ways we now know, MDRC. Here's a little summary list for you (don't say I don't treat you right):

- ◈ Self care is not selfish. It helps you look outwards.
- ◈ Treat yourself as you would a loved one.
- ◈ Picture your inner critic and say 'thanks but no thanks' or 'pipe down' as often as you need.
- ◈ Don't apologize for your every move, only if you truly owe an apology.
- ◈ Channel Beyoncé!
- ◈ Accept your vulnerability and listen to your needs.
- ◈ Learn to ask for help knowing you are loved.
- ◈ Find ways to move away from people-pleasing – because YOU ARE LOVED. And you are loved if people disagree with you.
- ◈ Learn to say no, you become more trusting and helpful.
- ◈ Consider the boundaries you need to conserve your energy and operate at your best.

God speed MDRC!

Interval

The image I had had of walking through that dark cave, picking treasures off the walls that I hoped might be practical ways to greet a healthier me at the end, was now feeling bizarrely real. The first half of the experience had given me the time and knowledge to understand my holistic diagnosis. Not just that Lyme disease, viral load and immune dysfunction can put the brain into a chronic stress response so the body can't heal, but the (frankly stunning) revelation that some seemingly innocuous, everyday life choices had also been bad for me and had overwhelmed my stress pot. It was extraordinary that my hunch had been right – the ways I had been living, often unknowingly, that had trapped me from being my true wild self, had genuinely had an impact on my body.

It truly made sense that being my wild self meant living a bold, adventurous, uniquely purposeful life; not stuck in conventions and rules that caged me and my inherent identity; not bound by limiting beliefs, lack of self-expression and connection; not trapped in fear to ask for help or state boundaries. Now, five treasures in, my longings were changing to become about those things – belonging, surrender and trust, acceptance, self-compassion and kindness. Here I was in the middle of the metaphorical cave, and what felt like literally halfway through my life, awake to who I was and what was important to me, in a whole and true way for the first time.

The second half seemed like it was going to be about reclaiming my unique identity. To learn how I tick as I considered being able to go back into the world again. That made sense to me because, as we can all hopefully agree, MDRC, self-compassion and love mean choosing to be on your own side. And to be on your own side, you need to know yourself. How can you love someone without knowing them? In serendipity, I happened upon something thrillingly vital for me to learn about my unique identity.

I knew that I was an introvert and at times an extroverted introvert – which was invaluable information to manage myself well. But I also fell into another category: I was a highly sensitive person (HSP). Oh, the joy of reading about it. Never felt so seen! I shall explain forthwith.

One in five human people are highly attuned and sensitive. It's the same across the animal kingdom. Those people with the trait are vital to help the community survive. I see us as the meerkats of the bunch: we would have popped up on sensing the faintest noise or smell in caveperson days to alert the extroverts – who were probably having an admin meeting or cooking in a busy kitchen, or just down the pub chatting – that danger might be nearby. Without us highly attuned beings, you'd all die! You're welcome.

Obviously we don't live in caves any more (never say you don't learn from me), but HSPs are also the ones who can tell when someone is suffering, and often take on important advisor roles in society. Clinical psychologist Elaine Aron, who coined the phrase (I highly recommend her book if you think you or a family member might be an HSP), says:

[HSPs] are the writers, historians, philosophers, judges, artists, researchers, theologians, therapists, teachers, parents and plain conscientious citizens. What we bring to any of these roles is a tendency to think about all the possible effects of an idea. Often, we have to make ourselves unpopular by stopping the majority from rushing ahead. Thus, to perform our role well, we have to feel very good about ourselves. We have to ignore all the messages from the warriors that we are not as good as they are. The warriors have their bold style, which has its value. But we, too, have our style and our own important contribution to make.

Yup, it's official, we help the human race survive. Again, you're welcome. It takes a village ... We *all* matter and have value.

It was so vital to get this 'diagnosis' (it isn't a disorder or a condition, just part of who we are) because it requires management. This big, noisy world is pretty overstimulating for an HSP, and empathy overload is definitely a thing. As the internet meme goes:

Friend: 'Wanna hang out tomorrow?'

Me: 'I actually performed an activity yesterday. Please wait the three-day recovery period to submit another enquiry.'

No wonder my body couldn't recover without having boundaries; I needed my energy levels to be managed so expertly.

Many people, not realizing they are HSPs, feel as though they just don't fit into their culture (a bit like me in a nightclub). As Elaine Aron says, 'Because we don't fit the ideal model of recent society, we have to love ourselves intently.' And indeed, we all do.

As we get to know ourselves more, we can be our own best cheerleaders, ignoring the inner (and outer world's) criticism and rejection. (Shall we play some heart-swelling music?) With that, I was ready to sashay into the second half of the cave and my newly bolstered life, singing 'Getting to Know You' from *The King and I*, swinging my hips with gay abandon like I do at zebra crossings. Do come with . . .

Treasure Six

Why We Do What We Do

TREASURES PICKED UP: Integrity, meaning, purpose, nurturing your unique gifts and skills, value-based living, being over doing

PATTERNS SMASHED: Success, status and achievement focused, pressurized career path, busyness and overworking

WATCHWORD: Goodness

SOUNDTRACK: 'Heigh-Ho' from *Snow White and the Seven Dwarfs*

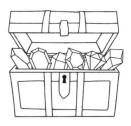

Why We Do What We Do

Off To Work We Go

My home had become a place of refuge in illness. I made different 'zones' to 'do' illness as well as I could. There was the cosy armchair that looked out on to the little garden to watch the birds. From there I sipped from my favourite tea mug and mindfully savoured some dipped-in dark chocolate. It was also a comforting place to practise breathing exercises (when I had the self-control to do so). There was the Lego table near the fire. From there I . . . well, I did Lego . . . I invested in an extra-long, super-king bed (hello to any fellow giants that know the necessity) which has the comfiest mattress I've ever known – like sleeping on a cloud (I imagine – I've yet to sleep on a cloud). And I created a, what I call, 'day nap and exercise area', where I would do some stretches or gentle tai chi moves. I was doing illness as well as I could; I failed every day in some way, of course, but that's okay. I was slowly reducing the stress in my pot.

It was all contributing to my new-found sashaying energy that made me eager to consider my place outside the confines of a sickbed. I wondered whether it was time to create a zone for work. I was by no means out of the woods and back to all cylinders firing, but brain fog was lifting (which felt like a miracle), light sensitivity had entirely gone (it had meant

227

months of drawn curtains until early dusk so this too felt miraculous), reading was less exhausting and writing seemed a possibility. I felt a flutter of excitement at the thought of being able to get back to some work. Was it time to consider writing a new comedy script? A couple of producers had asked whether I would adapt some books for film. I'd had to frustratingly decline, but maybe I was ready to sashay to my email inbox and say I would now be happy to talk about it. Plus, how wonderful it would be to have meaningful distraction.

I had missed work so very much. And I loved the idea of going back with a healthy, rounded attitude to it from all I had learnt, and all I was still learning, about how I uniquely tick. Was it time? As if to signify to my brain that it was, I did a little march and a skip to go off to work, humming the Disney classic: 'Heigh-Ho . . .'

Get Out Of Your Home But Stay In Your Home

What a woman who has started to sashay and skip – on considering working again after many years – doesn't need is a global pandemic. Does anyone, at any time? (I hasten to add, I'm not being flippant about Covid, MDRC. It was utterly horrendous for so many people, for so many reasons, and even though it caused significant health setbacks for me, I am aware I was one of the lucky ones, and my heart goes out to anyone still reeling from the front lines.)

It was a strange time in my story because I'd been advised, based on the remaining cluster of symptoms I still had, including some remnant fatigue (which meant, frustratingly, some aspects of my work were still not possible), to consider mould poisoning as one of the reasons my immune system might still be dysfunctional. Mould poisoning?! I'd never heard of such a thing. I was absolutely sure that couldn't be the case, but the inflammation levels in my body were high enough to warrant investigation. I was waiting for results from something called a 'dust swab' on my house – a testing of dust to assess air quality and toxin levels. I was told that if the dust swabs came back highly toxic, it would be wise to move out. This was happening at the same time that news of Covid was rolling in through our airwaves, and the threat of something called 'lockdown' loomed. If that became a reality, well, it was going to be illegal not to be in your own home. A couple of weeks went by and I was in complete denial of either lockdown becoming a thing as 'surely Covid was just going to be like flu' (remember that lovely initial naïve hope?), or mould poisoning being something real or serious that could affect me.

And then the results came. On both fronts. The toxicity levels of mould in my house were ten times the level the World Health Organization stipulates as acceptable, and I was advised to get out as soon as possible with just the clothes on my back and a few essentials . . . but in two days we would be in lockdown and I had to stay in my house. I was in shock. My own home, which had become my place of refuge, was part of what was making me sick, and I had to get out quickly before it became illegal to leave. I spent a very shaky day on rental sites wondering where to go and how to make it work. Until luckily I thought of a friend who was abroad, couldn't get back and might let me stay in her house. She did. Thank God for kindness.

With the gift of a roof over my head, I actually found that first lockdown to be a joyous couple of months. I remember feeling guilty about that as I saw the devastation around me. But I know most people housebound with an energy-reducing illness will tell you they experienced the same joy. For the first time we felt a lift in the daily grief of disappointment in all we longed to be able to do, those things that (healthy) others might take for granted. I didn't have to be sad about missing out on a roast lunch in a pub, or a picnic, or a birthday party, or a cuppa in a café, or a holiday, or, well, anything. They didn't exist for those few months and the relief was immense. Suddenly others had an insight into a housebound status and what missing out on the basics of life, that they hadn't realized were quite so wonderful and vital, was like. We were not alone in the disappointment. And people were more available to talk and FaceTime. We were literally not so alone too.

The thing that surprised me though, MDRC, was that I was also utterly relieved by the fact that most work was not an option. Odd, when I had been excited about getting back to it. But it showed me just how much pressure I'd been carrying about missing my job for so many years. I was so often judging whether my body was strong enough to go back, cross when it wasn't. It was work that I'd pushed myself to keep going for, before I collapsed again and surrendered. It was particularly painful that I had to halt work pretty soon after my first role in a Hollywood movie (*Spy*). I had worked so hard to get to a point of securing a lovely agent in the US, who was going to help me find more work as an actor, which felt like such a gift after writing and performing my own work for so long. Plus there was a game show remake in the UK.

Exciting possibilities that, in the end, I was never able to explore. I was pretty gutted, to say the least. I had been very envious of those who could continue to be in the industry I so loved and now, suddenly, with so many of us at home, all that disappointment was lifted.

It was a joyful lift. For a moment. And then in the spirit of being honest with myself, I realized, a little ashamed at first, that the hardest part of my life to let go of had been work. Did I value work more highly than things I know to be more important? Was it from work that I got my significance and worth? We often form our identities through it – we all need a job or role; developing and honing our skills is partly what helps us thrive; we all need to pay our bills; we might even feel that we are lost without work as it's such a key identifier. But if I was going to return with a healthy attitude, it couldn't be the thing that wholly defined me.

My job is more bizarre than many in that you 'get seen' in a way you don't with other jobs. The job is literally to be watched and stared at! (Though in my past office life I found ways to get moments of attention, like weighing my breasts to see how much they would cost to post. You're welcome, because I know many of you now want to try it . . .) I wondered briefly whether it was just because of the nature of my job that I found it harder to let go, but on speaking to others with a similar condition, it turns out that's not the case. One woman with chronic fatigue was a teacher, and she described feeling like she was clinging on by her fingernails not to have to resign. A huge part of her felt missing without her identity as a teacher. It's fascinating and strange that even when severely incapacitated with health issues, a grasping, pressurized need to get back to work can still exist. Surely stopping work is as innate an answer as not doing a daily bungee jump?

It seems to be yet another conditioned response. The idea that work has not only an extremely high (and often skewed) value but that we can sometimes feel like we only really exist, or exist at our best, with a job on the go. Without realizing it, work had become the biggest part of my life, and the loss of it was deeply felt. It was hard work to feel whole without, well, hard work. I had to admit that I felt lesser without it. I had been ready to heigh and ho, off to work I go, but first it was time to continue to learn my unique identity and how I inherently ticked. To make sure it wasn't work that made me feel complete as a person. This became the next treasure to lean into.

I knew God could move in mysterious ways but – get this, MDRC – I happened to discover that the lyrics to the Disney song I had been humming weren't about heading off to work but – wait for it – about coming *home* from work. Please say I am not the only one to have been duped into becoming such a productivity monster in this contemporary age that I automatically switched the lyrics?! I thought they'd been whistling and skipping excitedly off to work, and here I was confronting the concept of home as the most important thing. I didn't have a physical home to call my own, which made it all the more soul-searchy. I had no choice but to keep finding that home within myself, and who I was – without the external identifying me.

To work out who I was without work was a real gift.

232

The Wild

As you will have gathered by now, when I did get stronger and could go on small trips, it was nature I made a beeline for. And so, to ponder this work thing a couple of years after the mould and Covid debacle, I headed back to the Knepp Estate with its amazing rewilding project. There can't be a better place to contemplate 'human beings as over-productivity machines' than when surrounded by roaming, free wildlife whose existence is just to *be*. To survive, they have to be in the present moment. If they sit around to worry or contemplate, they die. If they don't follow their instincts, they die. Rather dramatic, MDRC, but my point is we're exhausting our wild, natural selves when we think productivity is the point of us. We are loved without providing any proof, just by being. Have we forgotten that work is not who we are? Strip away our jobs (many of us will leave or lose jobs for various reasons) and we are still the most important part of our wonderful selves.

I didn't know how much I had lost sight of that until a moment at Knepp. I was merrily going on a gentle walk (I will never, ever take a walk for granted again), thrilled to be moving with a little more freedom, delighted to be in fresh air, absorbed in the moment by the wildlife, when someone shrieked on recognizing me. That was fine, she was initially complimentary, and I made some lame joke that I might be her best wildlife spot of the day: 'The Miranda Beast'. She didn't really understand, which was awkward, but there wasn't time for a cringing silence as she hit me with this question: 'Have you retired, then?' My ego did a massive cartwheel. I got amusingly defensive to this poor, innocent woman: 'Um, no, I have *not* retired, thank you very much to you, just taken some time, had some stuff going on . . . and then there's been Covid, hasn't there, so you know . . . Retired? No, I'm here, look, hello. And my show is still on iPlayer, I'm here, hi, I'm relevant and things . . .' (I was close to pulling up my CV online and reciting a monologue.) We all have an ego to varying degrees, but my reaction was strong enough to make me consider my identity had, at least in part, become wrapped up in work.

Blimey, MDRC, I just looked up from my laptop (I am writing this section from, once again, Knepp) and was confronted with an extraordinary sighting of wild in this wood. A kestrel swooped down to pick something off the grass, and, to get my heart racing, a very large red stag walked slowly in front of me, taking an unnervingly long time to stare and check me out (it's rutting season so he's full of testosterone and I didn't want to fall victim to random stag rage or indeed urge!). I'm in a busy, human-swarmed patch of Southern England and could have been rammed by a stag and pecked by a kestrel. But what wonderful wildness to witness. I want to be that free and at home with myself, with no specific role or job to define me, feeling majestic despite someone thinking I have retired! To just be. Is that really possible? To get to a place of letting what we do be only part of us, an act of service, a way to pay the bills, small steps towards a dream perhaps? Not forging a career or being under pressure to 'get ahead'. Not fearing the outcome, just working as part of being. Couldn't I just be like that stag and wander around a wood and occasionally kill or rut something? (That was an analogy. Please don't worry about me.)

When did work become about status and significance? Shouldn't it be about a 'why'? A why based on values beyond a notch on the CV? The red stag didn't need a LinkedIn profile to prove himself. Possibly getting a little obsessed with the stag . . . If we take the pressure off work as a career or accolade and make it about doing some good and helping improve the little patch of the planet we live on, don't we feel some release? Certainly when I thought about dolloping some goodness on my patch (sounds weird) while I was recovering, it made confinement due to illness a lot easier. It started to halt any lurking fear of insignificance. *Just plop bits of goodness about*, I thought!

When I came across author, researcher and speaker Simon Sinek and his work on 'Finding a Why', it became the nub of this treasure (lovely word, 'nub'). That was what this time was going to be about. Finding my why. Simon Sinek says that having a why and a mission statement is not just for businesses but individuals too. It's our purpose, cause, what we believe in. Examples I found include Spotify, whose why is 'to unlock the potential of human creativity by giving a million creative artists the opportunity to live off their art and billions of fans the opportunity to enjoy and be inspired by it'. I mean, that would get me up in the morning if I worked for Spotify (though I appreciate most companies have issues we don't always love). A charity I came across during lockdown called Astriid has a beautiful why: 'Helping people with long-term health issues and their carers find meaningful employment so that the routine and sense of normality can provide a greater sense of well-being.' Simon Sinek's why as an individual is 'to inspire people to do the things that inspire them, so that, together, each of us can change our world for the better'. Our why is about who we are not just what we do. It can sound rather grand to declare your own personal mission statement, but reading Simon's, I could completely see that if he lost his job, he could still work towards his why in his everyday life – in conversations, encouraging young people; it would be a filter for choices from volunteering to the kind of movies he might like to watch. He is fired up when people are inspired. Simon says that when he found his specific why, he stopped talking about what he did and started talking about what he believed. He said it changed his life to start with a why and to live his life with purpose, on purpose. Yes please, I'm in.

There are ways to work out how to hone your why, if you so desire, MDRC (Simon has an online course, for example). And you don't ever have to share it with another soul if you don't want to. Considering I have shared quite a lot with you so far in this book, I will tell you what mine began as. Mainly as it was writing the book that made it clear (the why for the book, I suppose) . . .

To help people see who they are beyond the world's rules and pressures and their own pasts. To set people free to be who they are made to be, so that the world is healthier and happier.

It does sound super grand (I am cringing a bit!). But I have to say, it made life instantly feel more exciting and fulfilling, in whatever job or conversations or tiny ways I might choose to use it. Yup, I'm all in. I'm off to prance with the power of a why like a wild stag.

Careers Advisor

To find any necessary patterns to smash, I went back to the beginning to uncover how the world may have caged me in on the work front.

I grew up in a culture where what people did, what their jobs were, was primarily what was acknowledged about them. To that end I was very much a child of the Thatcherite, individualistic, achievement-focused eighties (but, hey, we got Kylie and Jason . . .). And then there was the school system. I will never underestimate the privilege of an education, but some aspects of that system seem a little absurd, like the strict focus on academic results and what we want to aim for career-wise as early as aged thirteen or fourteen.

I was not remotely academically gifted or interested, and I wish I'd been told that our lives continue to unfold at their right pace after GCSEs; we all develop at different times and education comes to us in myriad ways throughout our lives. I wonder if the reason I had such bad hay fever on exam days was because my stress pot was bubbling over – taking said exam was not remotely close to my purpose – which is okay, there are many things we will have to do that we can't always file under our purpose. But in this case there was stress because of a sense I could be a failure if I, well, failed. You couldn't really fit me into a square hole academically – I was developing into a glorious round peg, thank you very much!

I remember I had a couple of sessions with a careers advisor. I filled in some forms and answered some questions, and she informed me what she thought was my best career option. In my first session, she told me she thought I was best suited to being a librarian. Let's just sit with that for a moment, shall we, MDRC? ME, a LIBRARIAN. (She was really not seeing my round peg.) At the time I had very little interest in reading. I listened to audiobooks to try and get through exams, and York Notes were very much my friends (life does develop – no one at school would have thought my writing a book would make any sense at all). I mean, there are so many things wrong with me being a librarian, but can we just imagine me sitting quiet *all day*? In fact, no, that's not quite right. In the spirit of getting to know myself – I'm happy being quiet all day, I like days to myself. But imagine me staying quiet all day when I am told to be quiet all day. If I'm told to maintain any sense of decorum, I must immediately make a fart noise. I would have spent all my days as a librarian plotting how to make noises and then search around, mastering the look of 'What was that?' I would have taken my clothes off at least once a week and gone up to someone as if nothing was out of the ordinary and ask them in a whisper if they needed help. In fact, ideally, I would have been asked for a book when fully clothed and then returned fully naked with the book. Just to see if they'd say something or scream – and if they did, I would have gone 'shush' in their face. There's just too much comedy to my being a librarian. It would have been a red rag to a bull (or stag). Plus, I wasn't even doing English A level or reading a book at the time!

Having lost all respect, I confess, for my careers advisor, when I returned for my second visit, having been told to come with some reflection on her suggested career for me, I was extraordinarily juvenile. I told her that I didn't think librarian-ness was right for me but that I felt I had a calling as some interests were coming to mind. She was excited and intrigued. The game was to get her to say, 'I deduce you want to be a baker,' so I started listing things like, 'I love early starts. I like flour. I love the smell of biscuits. I don't mind crumbs in the bed . . . I don't know what it's all pointing at . . . I am a big fan of Josephine Baker.'

She wasn't amused. I can't think why she didn't think I was destined for comedy!!

'. . . And What Do You Do?'

After school, it's not long before we're going to social functions where we shall undoubtedly get asked the challenging question: '. . . and what do you do?' Why is it that after learning someone's name, it's often the first thing we ask? Obviously, there's the obligatory 'Where did you come from?' that can slip in first – with or without a discussion on traffic and specific A-roads travelled. But then soon comes that penetrating, piercing almost accusatory '. . . and what do you do?' It's as if this is your chance to prove yourself. To signal whether it's worth continuing to chat to you, or whether they should move off to another, more interesting and dynamic person. I have friends in their fifties who still fear that question. And, indeed, will even avoid a social event because of it. People shudder at their worth being evaluated.

As Parker J. Palmer wrote in *Let Your Life Speak*: 'The deepest vocational question is not "What ought I to do with my life?" It is the more elemental and demanding "Who am I?

What is my nature?"' I love that he says it's the more demanding question. It's easier to be labelled a success, or aim for
success, and ignore who we really are. But – it's not 'I am
what I do', it's 'I do what I am'. Ooh, bit profound, MDRC, but I
like it!

Getting to know The Boy from Bristol while I was writing
about this was fascinating timing. Because he didn't give a
rat's arse (his words) what I did for a living. In fact, on any
occasions we did talk about my work, we would laugh about
how little he had seen of it (RUDE). If a show with me
popped up, he would switch off pretty quickly as he didn't
want to know the person on the TV. It was such a gift to
have someone say it was the real me that they wanted to
know, and to be complimented on aspects of myself I might
have forgotten. That gift was more important than any
fleeting moments of self-worth created by sitting in a make-
up chair and having a photo shoot. I will always keep
stamping on the fame myth, MDRC. You can't success your
way to self-love.

The fact that '. . . and what do you do?' has become a
phrase synonymous with initial social interaction – and, more
to the point, that we have a fear of or a pride in answering
it – is perhaps an indicator many of us are on the merry-go-
round of believing our worth comes from what we do.

Isn't the interesting question 'Why do you do what you
do?' That's when you see the real person, their passion and
inspiration. Simon Sinek (aka Mr Why) says passion is
output – you can't force a passion upon someone; it's their
true self-expression and what makes hard work and

sacrifice worth it. With a passion behind what you do rather than a pushing to do something you are not passionate about, you also have far more resilience to stress. There it was, a big clue for making sure work doesn't add too much to the stress pot.

The Success Trap

The desire – or need – to prove ourselves through what we do means that many people end up in a success trap. I couldn't help but think that the constant measuring and evaluating and judging of work success is no different to the inner critic's assault on our personal selves. It's not a kind or loving way.

I don't believe success is a bad thing. Sometimes, it's simply a by-product of doing what we love. The trap is thinking that success is what makes us who we are, and that success can be a bedrock for happiness. A 'why' is about something other than achievement and measurement. Think about it, MDRC. If someone's why is to get fame, they're always going to be terrified of losing it; if a person's why is 'to be the best', they're always going to be under enormous competitive pressure, and compare themselves to others.

I read an interesting book called *Humankind* by Rutger Bregman. He was thought-provoking in stating that we have become more and more out for ourselves and our personal gain. Our focus is no longer on friendship, community and spiritual things but on the trap of achievement. But – and this is a game-changer – our goals are never going to make a difference unless the value *behind* them is to make a difference. I was buoyed, MDRC. I thought about how nicely this connects with learning to love ourselves never being a selfish act. For as we learn to get to know ourselves in this way (with our whys), we might just find that we have an impact on the community around us. Dolloping our goodness around the place!

But that's quite enough about doing good for the wider world. Back to me! I was in a very unusual situation – it's not often that one finds oneself so long out of the world. I continued to be able to stand back and see just what the rat race was doing to my nearest and dearest, and it all seemed completely mad. Frenzied. I became tense as friends told me about their working lives. Not many seemed to love and feel fired up about what they were doing. The need to be constantly available had clearly become worse. I would hear things like, 'I'm exhausted but I should go to this event because then I will be seen to be a team player.' An endless sense of having to prove and keep up. All the carrying on carrying on in all its messiness. I worried about my friends. I was not witnessing people skipping to work, neither were they skipping back; instead they were limping their way home.

I concluded that the only way to make work a healthy, functioning aspect of ourselves came down to working out why we do what we do. Which paradoxically makes it much easier to dare to knock on doors, go to job interviews, start the first day of a job, because it's not entirely about our evaluation, how we move up and onward, it's about the way we bring some good into that workspace. That would surely take some of the fretting and striving off. It might also make it easier if we are stuck in a job we don't love, or working within a company we don't respect, as we remember our why is *ours*, who we are, what enlivens and inspires us, and can be applied in small ways to all parts of our day. When I was data inputting in my twenties in an office, it didn't particularly excite me, but I look back and see that I was actioning my 'why' outside of work, with suggestions for fun at lunch break or hosting activities when we clocked off. I think back to the art of gathering from Treasure One and how hosting is a great arena to fulfill our unique 'whys'. I really hope that if I ever went back to data inputting, I would be able to reframe it. Instead of focusing on how I perceived it (i.e. as a boring job), I would be able to see that it was helping others to be freed, because the company needed that efficiency to run smoothly. Stamp your 'why' on the mundane and those tasks might come alive and even be rewarding.

I remember speaking to the project manager looking after the renovations on my house – the man who de-moulded me (steady . . .) I asked why he'd taken the project on, as the whole mould thing was rare and therefore a little complicated. He replied, 'On hearing about your health problems and knowing the building industry, I felt I wanted to do my best for you and protect you.' Talk about a dollop of goodness. (And I won't lie, I did swoon.) I don't know whether he was loving his job or whether it was a grind, whether it was financially rewarding or he was scraping by, but it was clear he knew he wanted to do it for something beyond that – to help another.

The Comedian Who Forgot They Were Making People Laugh

I was once backstage for a TV event after my fellow performer and I had had a difficult rehearsal, and we were feeling the pressure of the situation. We plonked ourselves down in a dressing room with a cold baked potato and a warm Diet Coke (classic BBC!) for our pre-show dinner and sat in nervy, tired silence until my fellow funny person said, 'Do you ever wonder why we do it?' I replied, 'Never.' 'Really?' was the searching reply. 'Never?' 'Never,' I repeated. 'So why do you do it?' they asked. I was surprised by the question. I thought my answer of 'never' would be implicit. I answered, 'To make people laugh, or should I say, to try and make people laugh.' 'That's the only reason you do it?' 'Yes,' I replied. 'Otherwise it all becomes a farce – please enjoy the pun.' There was a pause and then my fellow funny person, who was very well known in their funniness, said, 'Do you know, I have never thought of it like that?' 'Never?' I asked. 'Never.' I was amazed. I couldn't imagine being in comedy and that not being the clear mission (even if I had yet to hone my more detailed 'why' which encapsulates all parts of me). 'That changes everything,' they said. An energy came into the room from them – in that moment, they had a why. A slumped chest went to a strong, shoulders-back pose. The cold potato was washed down quickly with the warm Diet Coke and they put their head in the script with renewed vigour.

'You Can Do Anything You Set Your Mind To'

I know this is a phrase in common parlance that many people are inspired by. But as a piece of advice it has never really worked for me. I have always found it a pressure. So, when I came across these words from clinical neurologist Dr Caroline Leaf – 'You can do what you are predisposed to do with your genes and your skills' – I felt instantly calmer and encouraged. It felt an awful lot kinder, too. The way to love ourselves is *surely* to uncover and work on our unique skills and gifts. Going our own way, against worldly expectation and patterns, with our individual set of skills the world needs and wants is bold and brave. I think. And hopefully infinitely more satisfying.

It makes all the sense in the world for each person to have both a unique DNA and a unique set of gifts. Each only exists on this planet at this moment in history. You might just be the next great artist, politician, salesperson, inventor, train driver, human resources manager, nurse, farmhand, babysitter, writer, gardener, adventurer, fundraiser, parent, admin assistant, shopkeeper or zoo manager. Whatever you do matters. We're all inimitable, weird wonders with a point!

Get to know your gifts and nurture them, I say. That's a key route to finding your why. On which note, here are some fun tips I found along the way. Exciting, isn't it, MDRC?! Well, I'm fired up . . .

Remember What You Love

Remembering what you love might seem a rather basic idea, but it's such a cunning way to discover what may have become absent from your life. Thinking about what excites you and your inherent passions unlocks the stressing and striving brain and can help in rediscovering the real you, not the one who has worn a mask for years. Not the 'you' based on past conditioning.

All the 'ists' I read on finding our why said that we need to unlock the imagination in order to go back to the starting point of what we simply loved to do. Doesn't matter if it makes no sense, sounds childish, doesn't connect to a job – we can just allow our minds to wonder. The dots can be connected later.

I created my own list of questions. When I discussed these with friends, we had larks and genuinely made some discoveries.

1. **What did you want to be when you were younger and why?** I wanted to be a goalkeeper for the England football team. I was super emotional watching the Lionesses as in my youth, being a girl and playing football just wasn't a thing. It reminded me of my passion for sport and fitness, and women being free to be who they are (I was excited to capture that from the past and see where it might lead). I also remembered I wanted to be Joy

246

Adamson of *Born Free* fame. Who knows whether that's a thing or not . . . Doesn't matter.

1b. **If you were to go to a fancy dress party that said 'come as what you wanted to be when you were younger', what would you go as?** This was my own version of 1. I thought that when you dress up, you want to feel cool and excited and comfortable, so it might just unlock something. Or going to such a party might just mean the chance to stare at a lot of men in firemen's uniforms. Moving on . . .

2. **Tomorrow, you are going to be knighted or damed – congratulations! What is it in services to?** My answer was world peace via getting people galloping and laughing! One friend said 'saving orcas'. We all laughed. Guess what – she wants to do some volunteering to learn about them and how she can help. I mean, these larks can work.

3. **Write two or three sentences that you would want to be in your eulogy.** This came from a life coach who suggested I write my entire eulogy from the perspective of a friend, work colleague, family member and someone in the local community. It was embarrassing to start with, but when I realized only the coach would ever see it, I let rip (before I ripped it up) – and I was UTTERLY MARVELLOUS! The point being you can see themes emerging you may not have realized about yourself before. Plus it's fun to briefly be the most extraordinary human being that ever lived and a genius at every turn. . . .

4. **Who is your hero? And why?** There are reasons we admire people. Thinking about why might unlock

what you are passionate about and what values are important to you.

5. **You are ninety-nine. What are you telling your great-grandchildren or great-nieces or great-pets that you were brilliant at that might amuse and surprise them?** One friend said, 'I'm a really excellent driver.' It's so random what we come up with when we are just playing. But it helped her realize that there was part of her job she could do that would involve driving, which would help the company out.

6. **How would you like to have helped people?** My friend shouted, 'Make them not be extinct!' I had to calmly tell her she was still thinking about the orcas . . .

7. **What's an activity that even if you were feeling really exhausted and low, you think you might get up off the sofa for?** I put if Matthew Perry (RIP) came in the room to do a comedy scene with me. I also put 'hug a donkey'! Moving on . . .

8. **What do or did you naturally spend time doing, and time just flew by?** I spent hours playing all the parts in *Annie* in my bedroom after school. On having that memory, I ended up asking my agent if there were any productions of *Annie* around, or if he thought anyone would like to do one. There happened to be one on tour and they were wanting to come into the West End. I ended up having the chance to play Miss Hannigan. Crazy!

'You know how every once in a while you do something and the little voice inside says, "There. That's it. That's

why you are here . . ." And you get a warm glow in your heart because you know it's true? Do more of that.' – Jacob Nordby

I love that quote because the success trap can so often mean we lose that feeling. Many may never have felt it. Which is why I think it's cool that remembering what you love ultimately leads to dreaming. It is often said that if you have had any time of crisis, when you start to dream again it's a sign you are coming back to yourself – I have certainly seen it of mid-life friends with empty-nest syndrome or ending a lifetime of work or going through a divorce.

When I was very unwell someone said to me, 'If your symptoms and your situation just evaporated, what would you do?' At the time I couldn't imagine or answer that. I knew I needed to dream again. I since learnt that by dreaming of the things that bring us joy and meaning and excitement, we are telling the brain we are not in fear, reminding it of possibility, which reduces the stress response and betters the immune system. Might as well dream!

Considering my why gave me glimpses into the 'new me' who could now be free from any past success traps, so that I could feel significant whether I stayed or got sicker, or ended up back on a film set. A dream job is not what we are searching for (some may never get their specific work dreams), but rather a why within our skills that is part of who we are. And dream big around that.

I will never stop dreaming and going towards what I love and what excites me. And I am sad my younger self was partly trapped in that arrivals hall because she thought she had to.

The Value Of Values

In perfect synchronicity I literally happened upon a book (I randomly found it under my bed) called *Dream Big* by Bob Goff, in which he first suggested taking some time to list out up to a hundred dreams, as improbable as you like. Then he said to put the dreams into categories – big, medium and small. It was thrilling. Sergeant Major Sandy loved it because it gave license to use a lot of stationery. There was flip chart paper, rulers, highlighters, coloured biros! I felt like a kid again. Dreaming was such a tonic.

Listing out small dreams was a genius suggestion because it meant the opportunity for meaningful excitements in the everyday. Great for all of us, but it meant even during severe illness there were ways to focus away from it and not keep my identity solely about being sick. Month on month my body noticed the increased verve! One of my small dreams was baking a cake (MDRC, I was soon turning fifty and had never done so). Incidentally, it provided a joyous date afternoon with The Boy. And I felt so freely myself that on having a hot flush from the ferocious mixing, without thinking and indeed without apology, I whipped my top off, popped the apron back over my bra and cracked on! And may I say the ferocious mixing was worth it – my first cake was a triumph. A moist lemon drizzle if you please.

Later in the book, Bob Goff tasks us to do an inventory of our dreams, culling those that lack meaning. That was a rude,

250

but brilliant, awakening. So many of my dreams were things that would be a lovely gift if I got to do them (dinner with the Prince and Princess of Wales; winning a BAFTA; playing tennis on Wimbledon Centre Court), but I was, as he suggested, the most excited about the ones that supported my values and could make a difference, help others, develop skills. No offence to your Royal Highnesses – I would still love to come over! But the point is, what would my daily activities be if that was my number-one dream – squats and lunges to perfect a curtsey? If I went on a film set with the aim to win a BAFTA, it would take all the joy out of creativity and camaraderie and my essential focus based on my why to connect with an audience. It would be absurd.

It was the first time I had so intentionally thought about value-based living. The psychologist Steven Hayes wrote a brilliant book called *Get Out of Your Mind and Into Your Life*. He says: 'Values are vitalizing, uplifting and empowering. Values are something you do, not something you *have*. If they are something you do, they never end. You are never finished.' Susan David, another psychologist and favourite 'ist', says in her book *Emotional Agility*: '"Walking your why" is the art of living by your own personal set of values.' It's values that get you up in the morning, give you that spring in your step. She says that with value-based living, you will wake up and get off autopilot and won't end up living someone else's life. Ooh, hello – I was certainly woken up to that. Especially when I saw that behaviours are affected by the beliefs, values and goals behind them.

I admit, MDRC, I was a little lost to know where to start to discover my specific values. I could only think of a handful of

251

value examples. So, I googled. (Value-based living surely needs to be part of education and careers advice.) Brené Brown's website came up, offering a list of values to peruse: creativity, love, helping, honesty, fun, change, peace, kindness, excitement, efficiency, order, fitness, faith, adventure, sustainability and on and on. It also offers a resource for how to hone our specific top two to five. There are other sites too – James Clear, Scott Jeffrey, and many more. Doing an inventory of my values was another game-changer in finding how I uniquely tick.

Here's a hot tip lest helpful MDRC, from 'ist' Dr Amen (a psychiatrist and brain disorder specialist). He uses a tool called the 'one page miracle' to clearly set out your values and goals in all aspects of your life. I considered it not just because it might involve using some fun stationery but because, he said – get this, MDRC – you have to tell your brain what you want. WHAT?! It's the number-one tip he gives to all his patients – you have to tell the front part of your brain that's involved in focus, forethought, judgement and impulse control what you want, what kind of person you want to be, how you want your relationships to be. Then every day you can see if your behaviour is working towards what you want. Amazing hack – amen to Dr Amen!

Also, as a little aside, I was bowled over when I learnt from 'ist' Christine Dunkley, an expert in dialectical behaviour therapy (DBT), a type of talking therapy, that often with people who are really struggling to get their needs met, she will suggest that instead of saying 'I need reassurance' or 'I need connection', they should state: 'I *value* reassurance and connection.' That then puts the power back on us and what we could do to reassure and connect. It's important to us, so perhaps we could reassure someone else or ourselves (we have such strength within, we may never know). I thought about all the nuance of boundaries and needs and having a busy thought life – but, if in doubt, follow the value. We are never going to get it right all the time, but values will always be the right guiding light to follow. Wow, this is really freeing.

Why You Are, Not How You Are

'Why do you want to get better?' When one of the specialists, or should I say specialist 'ists' (bit of fun), on brain retraining to reduce the chronic stress response said that to me, I knew it was important but considered it in some ways rather cruel. Did I need a reason? Don't we all desire good health to live life to the full? The 'ist' continued that without a clear answer to that question, it would be hard for me to do the daily tasks to recover. If you can start to remember who you are and why you want to be better, your focus can come off your circumstance and on to those visions. It became harder to sit on the sofa rather than doing the exercises to reclaim my muscle strength, for example. I understood it now. Everything becomes focused, intentional living with a why.

You have your reason to improve, get better, get up, change, keep going. You are loving yourself. If my value was to put a bit of goodness and kindness into the day, in whatever way I could, aligned with my why, then an ease would come. A smile on waking. A spring in my step. Life would feel possible and fun.

Discouragement and dissatisfaction come without a vision. As Nietzsche said (I just saw it on Instagram – that sounded like I have thumbed through all the world's philosophers): 'He who has a why to live for can bear almost any how.'

That was partly why work was something that would have been hard for me to let go of. We don't want to be in a rat race, but we thrive with meaningful work. That's why I loved discovering the charity Astriid, because their research shows that people, when they're unable to join in work life, struggle with their health. Human beings need meaning.

I am so grateful I had the time to think about why I work and my values. It will guide me until the day I die. It's not measurable, it's who I am. And it's who I am in every part of life. Who we are is more important than anything we do.

I was intrigued that many of the 'ists', including Simon Sinek, suggest that one way to discover your why is to listen to what any suffering in your life has led you towards caring about or opened your eyes to. As the beautiful quote from Frederick Buechner says: 'Your vocation in life is where your greatest joy meets the world's greatest need.'

I wasn't at a place I could believe that suffering always comes to good. But perhaps I was ready to consider that it doesn't all go to waste. I was struck that the values I needed at this time and wanted to live by were the watchwords of the treasures that had come from the darkness of illness so far: connection, faithfulness, peace, self-control, kindness and, from this treasure – goodness. Wow, For me, these treasures were more valuable than any Hollywood film career I had previously desired.

I was sashaying and skipping again. I was heigh-ho-ing, it's home from work we are go-ing. The things you can learn from a Disney song, eh?!

I did, too, eventually get back into my physical home – thank you to the mould man! It was time to make a zone in my house for some work within my limits, with a value-based why. (For what it's worth, MDRC, what came from that was an online shop called The Miranda Shop, which supports charities like Astriid and another charity that helps young people with difficult lives find work, Resurgo. Yup, maybe darkness doesn't all go to waste.)

Time To Tap In

Sometime later, I was watching an acting class. There was one exercise where the group stood on the outside around two players in the centre, and it was up to those on the outside to 'tap in' when they felt moved to have a go, swapping with whoever they tapped out. After the exercise the teacher was giving feedback and asked the few who'd never tapped in why they felt they hadn't. There was no admonishment for there had been no obligation for them to have done so. They said that they'd been caught up in the watching and the teacher gently encouraged them to listen deeper, privately,

255

as to whether there'd been any fear-based reason they might have preferred watching. Just because, as she astutely pointed out, sometimes we are in fear-based habits without realizing.

We do have to 'tap in'. Dreams aren't just for other people. Unique callings are for everyone, because they are unique! If one person can achieve a goal, feel like they have made a small difference, make a job change, then anyone can. It's not reserved for particular types of people. And some of the greatest change makers came from nothing. Where we start is not a barrier to how we can end.

There's nothing to lose by tapping in.

'What if you wake up some day, and you're 65, or 75, and you never got your memoir or novel written, or you didn't go swimming in those warm pools and oceans all those years because your thighs were jiggly and you had a nice big comfortable tummy; or you were just so strung out on perfectionism and people-pleasing that you forgot to have a big juicy creative life, of imagination and radical silliness and staring off into space like you were a kid? It's going to break your heart. Don't let this happen.' – Anne Lamott

Treasure Seven

Play

TREASURES PICKED UP: Joyful, fun, grateful, creative, spontaneous, curious, imaginative, adventurousness, wonder, pleasure

PATTERNS SMASHED: Seriousness, forgetting to play, fear of childishness, lack of movement, doing over being, ignoring nature

WATCHWORD: Joy

SOUNDTRACK: 'Into the Groove' by Madonna

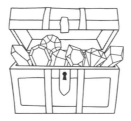

Play

'It's Time To Get Your Joy Back'

There was a little moment when I woke up one morning and found myself saying out loud, 'Right, Miranda, it's time to get your joy back; it's time to follow joy.' A tiny, and indeed strange, little moment. (I say strange but I probably talk to myself far more than I think – it can't only be me who finds themselves doing self-commentary: 'Need to get some peppercorns for that grinder ... Why is ground pepper less good and fun?', 'Does everyone take their phones to the loo?', 'Why am I in this room? I came in for a reason ... I'll go back and come in again ... Nope, still no idea ... ')

I knew this little moment was defining. I didn't feel like I'd lost joy *entirely* and I wasn't depressed. So where did this strong, definite voice telling me it was time to get my joy back come from? I was distracted from my pondering by a scuttling noise in the corner of the room. I feared it might be a mouse – I wasn't in the mood for dealing with a mouse. (Are we ever? It's hard to find joy in vermin.) But on daring to move towards the unnerving noise, I discovered a large butterfly flapping against an unopen window. Such a beautiful creature. The exquisite detail of its orange and white markings, the fragility and strength of its wings. The same thing happened, as it always does when I see any kind of animal in distress: I myself got distressed. This time it wasn't a panicky feeling, I just looked at it and said, 'Oh, dear thing, you look utterly bored and exhausted.' Exhausted by the fight to get out into its natural habitat, which it could see so clearly yet there was an impenetrable glass prison in its way; bored because it was in a room it was not designed to be in. It was designed to adorn, out there, in the world, under the expansive sky. I got a book and the butterfly seemed to gratefully step on to it and let me guide it to the other side of the room towards an open window. It didn't immediately fly away. It sat on the windowsill as if getting its breath back, its wings moving very slowly, testing to see what they had left in them. *How sensible*, I thought. *Don't rush to celebrate your freedom, just be there for now, gather your strength, let your difficult experience wash off you, and head out when you are ready. There's no rush, dear butterfly, no rush.* This, for the deft among you, was obviously about to become another metaphor! I was more distressed than normal for this dear creature because, on this particular day, I too felt exhausted and bored. I felt stuck and I wanted to escape. This must have been why I woke up saying, 'It's time to follow joy.'

I remember hearing that when cyclists train, they don't train to avoid potholes, they train to see the path between the potholes. If the drill was 'don't look at the potholes', their brain would focus on them, become fearful and inevitably go into them. Instead, they train to look at the clear path between the holes. Looking back – and this is why my firepit moment was so important for me – I can see I had become bored and exhausted because I'd spent years focusing on the potholes, overcoming the potholes, mitigating against the potholes, trying to control the potholes. I have said potholes too much now it doesn't seem like a word, and it's become sort of rude. POTHOLES!

When we are younger, playfulness and joy are naturally part of our day. We don't ruminate on the potholes of life because we're always looking for the next idea that gives us energy, creativity and fun. And we instinctively, literally and metaphorically, hop to it. Yes, that's partly because we have young bodies and less responsibility, but I believe all tired adults have felt a reprieve in moments of play. I had plateaued healing-wise, and that voice I woke up to was likely giving me the reason why. If we're constantly seeing life as full of obstacles to overcome, we can't but become exhausted.

I was living in a small way, internally flapping, agitated, like the butterfly trapped in the room. Thinking about dreams and values had given me more verve but the desire to get out and on with said vim and verve led to frustration. I could see life and all I loved beyond the glass. I was a wild creature who had snookered herself unknowingly. Even I – a silly creative who hated rules, who talked about setting people free – had become beaten down. Not just by recent illness, but because I'd fallen into yet another worldly trap – that play was not important. This was a startling realization, and woke me up to how much play had been eroded from my life. Joy, I hoped, would be another treasure on the way back to my wild self. Another gem for healing.

I was pretty certain what joy was, fundamentally. I knew the difference between fleeting happiness based on good life circumstances and internal joy that transcends any trappings we think might make us happy. I knew joy could be present even amid deep loss and sadness and difficulty. But I wanted to research to cement my understanding of it. And, joyfully, it was fairly simple. Well, joy wouldn't be boring or laborious, would it? Joy says, 'I'm here! Follow me, not the potholes, and you will find me.'

That was the first thing I learnt about joy. It's about the small moments. Little moments of joy subvert the ego and thinking mind that might be jealous of someone having a super-yacht because surely big, glitzy things like having a personal chef to provide constant canapés as one lounges on a front deck is joy? I know deep down those are examples of momentary happiness, if we experience anything remotely like it. (For me it would likely be a takeaway as I pretend the delivery came from my personal chef.) Otherwise all wealthy people would be telling us the 'answer to life' is their lifestyle, and then where would that leave the poverty in the world? No, that makes no sense at all.

Joy has to be about wonder. It's about plants and clouds and smiles and hot tea. And butterflies. It's about the every-day things. Not the awards, the exam results, the promotions, the bank balance. All those things are fleeting and finite. Joy says, 'Sorry, I couldn't care less about you being employee of the month, LOOK AT THAT PETAL IN THE RAIN – ISN'T IT AMAZING?!'

The thing about joy is that there will always be something akin to a petal in the rain to find in every moment. That's what joy feels like to me – grace. An unexpected gift that makes me smile despite it all. Something to be extraordinarily grateful for as I feel reassured and peaceful when basking in its pure and simple delight. I suddenly missed Peggy's soft fur – stroking a pet a noble example of joy as comfort.

The grace of joyful moments doesn't always feel quite so resonant without someone to share it with, and joy is always a deep connector, but there are times when we are alone, very alone, and so it's worth contemplating that joy is simply a reason for being. It feeds our soul. It's another part of who we are. That means joy is the ideas and dreams I have. From where I create. Laugh. Experience natural wonder. Feel a belonging (I found my fledgling faith gave me a surprising connectedness and joy). It's surely a key part of our identity? I read that even in the deepest grief, we need joy for a break on our nervous systems. It gives us the natural neurotransmitters and chemicals to mend tired brains and keep the negative bias in check. Healthy neurotransmitters are vital to build a healthy brain, which leads to effective immune and nervous system function. We need oxytocin, dopamine, serotonin, endorphins to survive and thrive, and they are produced when we play. Which is why children instinctively go to it. Science, rather thrillingly, continued to measure with the treasures. Following joy would be essential to regain a healthy body.

It was time to burn out remaining boredom and exhaustion. I was still waiting patiently on the windowsill to regain full energy, not yet ready to leap into work with my clear 'why', but my first and most important job was to follow joy (my joyb, if you will). To train my brain away *once and for all* from the potholes, and rediscover play as that was no doubt the portal to a lot more joy. I told you the treasure got more jolly!

Forgetting To Play

Whenever I'm asked if there was a moment when I knew I wanted to get into comedy, I have a very clear answer. I will never forget it. Which is unusual because I have an appalling memory (Lyme-type viruses tend to eat away at it – delightful) and this was when I must have been about eight. I distinctly remember watching Morecambe and Wise on TV and being absolutely mesmerized. Apparently (this bit I don't remember) I was open-mouthed looking very sombre as I sat quite close to the television on the floor, and my mother asked me if I was enjoying it as she hadn't heard a peep from me. I said, not taking my eyes off the screen, in a very serious tone, with a boot face, 'Oh, it's absolutely hilarious.' What I remember – and would explain my tone – was that I was captivated by the fact that I was watching two grown-ups being silly. There was such relief that came from seeing adults play, muck about and create laughter. It wasn't something to laugh about – it was a very serious matter! If there were ways to be silly and get laughs in this thing called the television, then I wanted part of it, because I couldn't bear to live in a world where I couldn't play and dance and sing and be a fool. That, to me, didn't seem like a life worth living.

This is a rather sad reflection on two things that all too often happen in life. Firstly, the times children are told, 'Shush, don't be silly.' Not that I blame any parent across the land for saying that sentence. Of course, when a child is being loud, or showing off, or repeating themselves over and over and over, any good parent is going to lose their patience at times and cry out, 'Just stop being silly.' I remember when a family member said it to me, and it was a seminal moment. One I am now grateful for. I couldn't understand why anyone would want to curtail my genuine joy. So, when I saw Eric Morecambe grinning at me down a television camera, I fell in love with him and with comedy.

The second reason my young self was bowled over by these two grown men clowning for my amusement was that seeing adults playing was obviously rare. My parents are fun-loving people and love a laugh, but if seeing Eric Morecambe meant an eight-year-old made a very serious decision to find play in her life for the rest of her days, she probably wasn't shown it very often by the busy adults around her.

I was rather taken aback when I read from an 'ist' called Stuart Brown in his book *Play* (the 'ists' are really good at book titles!) that his studies pointed clearly to joy being our birthright and intrinsic to our essential design. When you discover from an 'ist' that your hunch from your little life experience was correct, it's awesome and moving. I was even more shocked that my instinct was right when he said that 'for highly competitive, serious people, to realize later in life that they have missed this joy can be devastating'. I felt sure that must be part, if not all, of what makes up a mid-life crisis (whatever age that crisis might hit you). My point being it's when we realize that the so-called good and energetic *earlier* years have all been about building up aspects of ourselves in work, financially, finding a family, etc., to feel secure, or indeed being in constant service, has all been at the expense of joy. If joy is intrinsic to us, and play a way to get to it, is it no wonder we love to sing, to dance, to laugh, to skip, to cry at a movie ending, to read, to draw, to kick autumnal leaves, to build a snowman, to catch a wave, to laugh at someone falling over (as long as they don't hurt themselves!), to play catch, to make a daisy chain, to have a picnic, to ramble, to have sex, to lie down and look at the stars? Of course, losing those things could be devastating, only adding to our stress pot.

I wasn't surprised when Stuart Brown said that this happens because of the 'culturally supported idea that people who play are superficial, are not living in the real world, are dilettantes or amoral slackers'. If we're told at a very young age to stop being silly, then of course we're going to fear being playful in our thirties and forties and fifties. It's why people love getting older. It's then you hear, 'Oh, I've just given up caring what people think,' and you know they are free to start playing again. It's so loving to give ourselves joy.

My experience of losing joy was an ironic one. The memory of watching Morecambe and Wise aged eight on the floor of my parents' sitting room came back thirty years later, when I was sitting on the floor of my own sitting room, surrounded by a swarm of index cards with storyline ideas for my own comedy show. I was worried whether the episode was going to work or be even remotely funny – part of the unique pressure of a sitcom filmed in front of a studio audience (canned laughter is a myth in modern television). I was not a playful adult following their childhood dream with delight; I was a stressed adult, feeling the pressure of the job.

My personal sense of play had slowly eroded over the last two decades (it wasn't my job that was the cause). And I did indeed have a smouldering sense that something was missing.

I craved much of what I used to do for play, from those lovely school lacrosse team days, to long bicycle rides, to weekends with no other mission than finding a new picnic spot; and for years I wrote down 'dance classes' at the top of my New Year's Resolutions, knowing that it brought me so much joy to dance for no reason but to dance. Badly. And freely. I wanted to join a choir. I hadn't played tennis (one of my absolute top loves) for years. I wasn't in nature enough. The small and big things that brought joy had slowly disappeared from my life. It's not a good state of affairs if any of our jobs, roles and challenges mean we start to prioritize everything but play. But play being essential to my health was not something I'd learnt. I knew my life had lost some balance, but not the degree of the effects. (Another thing that I think should, without question, be on a school syllabus.) I wondered, with a tinge of sadness, how many of us have become unable to have time for the things we love.

But, like me putting dance classes on my list every year for over a decade, if we don't end up doing those things again, there's no need to beat ourselves up: we are doing our best and there's likely a deeper reason why. That's why I will keep saying forever – let's find those patterns we are in to smash them, to be able to do what we need to be freer, healthier and have the energy and meaning we want but may have lost.

Personally, I will not have the world telling me I have no time for joy or that if I am prioritizing it, I should 'stop being silly'. I know, for sure, that was one of the subconscious trappings I felt when I arrived at baggage reclaim – my daily play by nature of doing what I loved to do was instantly lessened as I got back to the 'real world'. I believe the world should be saddened and shocked when it realizes how little time we now have for play. As even my eight-year-old self watching comedy already knew. Which, for me, is more evidence that the wild self, innate in us, always knows the true way it needs to be.

What's Lazy?

The first pattern to smash is the fear of being perceived as lazy. How often I have noticed that people feel a pang of guilt for putting their feet up, sleeping in or having a nap, cascading into an apologetic ramble: 'Gosh, sorry, you must think me so lazy, I don't know why I'm so tired, can't believe I overslept, so unlike me.' We should be celebrating deep sleep, surely?! Have we forgotten that being tired and needing sleep is a normal part of human existence? Without sleep our bodies cannot repair from our daily activities. Personally, naps are my number-one top hobby!

Play is often what our best creatives and innovators and entrepreneurs do to release their imaginations; and play is what keeps us fit and inspired. What are we deeming as lazy, exactly? Why do so many people feel guilty for finishing work early to energize with a hobby or have a week on a sun lounger? Many don't take all their holiday leave . . . WHAT'S GOING ON?! It's so scary for us not to have any pause buttons. The fabulous Dolly Parton, as well as giving us the joy that is '9 to 5' (an absolute classic for a work dance break), said: 'Never get so busy making a living that you forget to make a life.'

The irony is that studies have shown that having a little moment of play in each day can not only make us happier but more productive. One study proved that animals that played more had a deeper developed cerebellum, which is the part of the brain responsible for key cognition. The more we play, the more our ability for attention and forward-thinking grows. If we are addicted to productivity, we'd want to play more. Ploughing on and on to get something done doesn't work.

There should be an award in corporations for the person who introduced the best game for their co-workers! My suggestion would be breakout orchestral conducting: as a piece of music gets piped around the office at random intervals, everyone stands and conducts with pens, pencils, rulers, chopsticks – whatever is on their desk. Really go for it! Please write in if you do this . . . I desire video evidence . . . I'd obviously also love to see any videos of people galloping in otherwise traditional or municipal building corridors!

Serious Business

I had such great bosses when I worked as an office manager and PA in the charity sector in my twenties. There was one amusing moment when our boss walked into the stationery cupboard to find three members of his admin staff sitting in chairs with damp hair, waiting for the fourth friend to cut our locks. He thought we were doing some necessary office supply inventory. In fact, we had set up a makeshift salon. He came in and said, 'Oh, sorry, finish up what you're doing and find me when you're done!' He knew we weren't taking the mickey (though perhaps sailing close to the line!). It was a very quick break, we'd make up the time. He knew that we would be back at our desks with smiles on our faces (and good haircuts), ready to work with renewed vigour. We loved what we did, we liked what the organization stood for (it had a why), we could dig in and do the mundane, and happily. But we needed to break out and play. We were a group of twenty-somethings not yet ground down by responsibility or fearing being deemed unserious or lazy. Probably because we weren't defined by our jobs.

One factor in losing my joy was when I started to get serious about my work, viewing it as a career. I think it was part of the turning-thirty nonsense – that strange convention by which we all feel at thirty we should be in some ways important and clearly established, and then grip on to 'success'. Jobs will have stressors and pressures and take up huge chunks of time. That can't be avoided. But with a 'why' and a balance of joy, the stressors can be part of the job and not detrimentally draining. We may have a job we want to master and need to invest in, but pressure grows because we drop joy. What a terrible example to show our children, don't you think, MDRC? We are feeding into them that adult life is only about doing, over-stretching to become very 'serious' and 'important'.

I tell you what's very serious about work – not playing.

Not just the vital health benefits. I felt sure I wouldn't be alone in wanting to be remembered for bringing some bubbliness to work and life? The things I will remember about my colleagues are not the scenes we did, not the mastery at their job, fine as it was, but the behind-the-scenes malarkey. Them, just being them. And if it was a playful moment, that will always be the first and most cherished memory. Although the moment I came into a rehearsal solely wearing three well-placed promotional stickers for the play we were doing might be one my colleagues desire to forget . . . Moving on . . .

'Don't Be Childish'

I was intrigued to see that in the spirit of letting masks down with The Boy from Bristol (MDRC, I could deny the frisson no more, and didn't shy away from continuing to rendezvous with him), the guard of silliness was one of the hardest. Probably why I showed him the Lego and I baked a cake half-naked, because I wanted reassurance about the fear of ever being over-the-top or childish. That can but be a culturally conditioned fear.

I think women certainly have been led to believe that expressiveness in the form of childish joy is not something to behold, and a partner would desire somebody a little more sophisticated. WHAT NONSENSE IS THIS?! What was I to do – don a bonnet and recite something on the pianoforte? When I was as silly as I naturally wanted to be, it led to the best moments. When we laughed the most. When we connected the most. Because play is wild, it cannot contain a mask. If it does, it's not play.

It seems wrong that we say to older children and young adults, 'Don't be childish' (the next sting up from 'Don't be silly'). I asked my niece once what her favourite time of day was. She said the evening, and I agreed, 'Oh yes, me too, because it's bedtime and we can start to relax.' She looked

273

confused and replied, 'No, because I'm so excited about the next day.' I had to admit, with a heavy heart, that at the time I was struggling with lack of energy and I was rarely excited about the next day. That hit hard – we can never have the same day twice. Each day is so precious.

Shouldn't we be so humble as to learn, or relearn, from the young? They should be turning around to us: 'We're not being childish. We're playing because it's the best part of the day and really good for us, please, you need to join in.'

Just For Pleasure

In moments of energy (occasionally flitting off the windowsill to test my wings) and reconfiguring how to do life after such absence from 'the norm', I had an unusual question to solve. I understood we need meaning, to feel some sense of achievement as we follow and use our skills, but my reverberating question was: So, pleasure, just pleasure – is that okay? Is that part of it all – just to be, have some fun, without clear purpose? I genuinely found myself asking that (before I fully dismantled the 'need to justify our existence' myth).

The answer is . . . drumroll . . . this will come as a massive surprise within this treasure . . . YES. The answer is yes, yes and yes. Absolutely blooming yes. And all the yeses that can be collected in the Kingdom of Yes. If the linchpin upon which everything unlocked in my research was loving and looking after yourself, then how could we possibly stop giving ourselves pleasure? It's what joy wants for us. Doing enjoyable acts just for the fun, to show we matter, has an extraordinary impact on our holistic health. However small they are. We may yet be in a place of being able to laugh regularly. And that's okay. Without Treasure Three (Feel, Grieve, Let the Past Be the Past), going through and feeling what I needed to feel, I may not have found the emotional range to get to a joy that meant I was reunited with my wheezy laugh and gummy smile. And oh golly, wow, the power of laughter. Pure grace from joy's fountain. It was worth finding the way back there despite any grief I had to endure. It's one of the greatest gifts of my life to be able to laugh until my ribs ache.

Get this from 'ist' Dr Caroline Leaf: laughing is often referred to as 'internal jogging' . . . a really good belly laugh can make cortisol drop by 39 per cent and adrenalin by 70 per cent, and increase endorphins (the 'feel-good' hormones) by 29 per cent.

Wow, wow and thrice wow! When we do things just for pleasure we are enlivened, and our stresses and strains are eased. Yay – let's take the stress out of our pots!

Also, genuine fun fact alert: even fake laughter has the same effect, which is why 'laughter yoga' is becoming popular, and brain retraining experts for chronic conditions suggest that even saying 'ho, ho, ho, ha, ha, ha' helps the body, and often leads to real laughter. You can feel ridiculous but hey, if it works, it works. Double fun fact: the reason it works is because – GET THIS – the brain doesn't know the difference between what is real and what is imagined. WHAT?! MIND-BLOWING. More anon . . . Back to pure pleasure . . .

I say let's not wait until we're retired for such fun. Surely, we want to jump and gallop before our pelvic floors force us to stop and we've missed the moment! (Side note: I learnt that bouncing is good for the immune system – licence to trampette and trampoline fully granted.)

We're more likely to get to retirement age if we keep playing. Plus, I've always thought that a lot of so-called fun 'retirement-age activities' should be acceptable and partaken of in younger years. Who says bingo is for the over-sixties? Not me. I went often in my twenties! Best nights ever. Not only because I got sausage and mash for £1.50. Not just that. Really not. I've had the best fun in aqua aerobics that was supposedly for over-sixty-fives, I've always loved crafts, and I love the idea of a slow-paced, non-bouncy, quiet dance class in which farting as we move is accepted (possibly followed by a glass of sherry and then getting a bit bossy). Retirement is wasted on the old!

It's in our inherent design to experience and partake in pleasure. We'd be a fool not to be a fool, MDRC.

Get Into The Groove

When I did eventually get around to doing a dance class in my thirties – sadly, a pumping, throbbing, loud-music kind of a class, with people treating it as much as a workout (I wanted to hone my inner dancer craft . . .) and looking at themselves adoringly in the vast mirror (even the person wearing flesh-coloured Lycra . . . Bold – you go, girl!) – my inner critic had an absolute field day. I knew it probably would because it had taken me years to dare to go to a class. It told me I was too unfit, too tall, too goofy to go (Pipe down, Sandy!). It convinced me I was safer at home, working or watching TV. As I believed the inner critic, before I knew how to challenge her, I noticed that I slowly became more inhibited. I was awkward doing a dance routine at work, wanting to reduce it to something small and insignificant. I didn't get up at a friend's house and freely galumph around when a piece of music moved me to do so. My inner critic won for a bit. It's ridiculous to me now, I'm pleased to say. But it reminds me that if we don't stand up to our past bullies, then that criticism oppresses our inner child. We will start to feel less of who we are. And do less of who we are.

Let me explain the term 'inner child', lest you think I've gone therapeutically severe on you. When I heard that term I was alarmed – I feared it might mean going to a kind of therapy that makes you sit opposite a small empty chair to imagine your younger self and talk to it. I know that sort of approach is used and can work wonderfully, but I also know initially I would be hampered by finding it weird. I think I would suggest to the therapist that my inner child had just told me that she desperately needs a Twix – 'It's not me, it's her, I promise you.' – so I could run out and, well, buy and eat a Twix . . . Luckily the 'ists' explained the concept of the inner child relatively simply. All hail the 'ists'.

Ready, MDRC? The inner child can be described as a part of our subconscious that has been picking up messages before it was able to process them mentally. It holds emotions, memories and beliefs as well as hopes and dreams. That's why we remember with joy what we wanted to do when we were younger. That's why we remember the smell of freshly cut grass when having a picnic with our grandparents. It's the part of me that has an inexplicable emotional reaction to the smell of the cleaning products in the old sports club. Our inner child is very important because all those excitable, happy and most importantly safe memories we cherish – they are a signpost to what we could lovingly give ourselves now. Everything is healed in safety. As we create more of those kinds of experiences, we invigorate and can heal our worn-down, even traumatized, adult selves who can be shown that now is a different time, with no threats of the past. Now, we are nurturing and loving ourselves with the things we had forgotten we loved and needed. I find that so beautiful.

If a loss of play resonates with you, I can truly recommend making space for activities to nurture and heal that inner child (even if it's two minutes in a day). Go on a bicycle ride, sit under or even climb a tree, draw a rabbit! Anything that lights you up and makes you feel safe. It all shows your brain you are doing things in a new way. A little warning: aliveness and spontaneity from the inner child is exactly what the inner critic does not like. They want us to behave and be sensible – anything not to risk being told off. If that critic pipes up, that doesn't mean you are on the wrong path. Tell it to very much pipe down and keep going, MDRC.

(Side note, MDRC, as regards dreaming, which following joy can lead to. I am blessed to find it easy to dream big, but it's very normal for the inner critic to pop its little head up with a, 'Who on earth do you think you are to consider such a grand idea for yourself?' Imposter syndrome might try and take a bite at you. There's sometimes a need to undermine the fear of being misunderstood. Or the fear of what people think. It is hard to be unique when you are comparing, and assuming judgment from others.)

That first dance class I went to was nerve-wracking. I stayed at the back. I wore very baggy clothes. Each week I took the next step in challenging the inner critic. Wearing a t-shirt without a baggy sweatshirt, then leggings instead of tracksuit bottoms, then moving to the centre of the back line a little closer to others. Just very slowly, keeping that sense of safety at all times. That critical voice might always be with us to a certain extent, but if we can laugh at it, and do things despite it, we're free.

I can't wait to get my fitness back and get to a dance class. I'd probably be second row, good view of myself and the teacher in the mirror, leggings and a singlet (whatever the bingo wings are doing), just going for it. Pretending I'm a combination of Ginger Rogers, Flavia Cacace and Darcey Bussell. In fact, when I go on tour again, I'm blooming well going to do a tap dance. Why? Because I can't! But because I'm free, and that's more important . . .

What Is 'Play' Exactly?

After understanding some patterns I needed to smash, it helped me to get a clear definition of play to start to put that specific quality back into my life. It might be easy to think playing means bouncy castles and ball pools. To me, the more of those for adults the better, but no, play has a science behind it. Stuart Brown (the 'ist' I call Mr Play) informs us that play, which children teach us perfectly, consists of seven key things. As it's the playful treasure, I shall write a little listicle. In French and Spanish. I know, what a thrill. De nada . . .

1. **Uno. Play is done for its own sake. It's not about purpose or achievement.** It's not play if you are at a tennis club furious for missing a volley because you want your hands on a trophy.

2. **Deux.** It's voluntary. It's something that you long to do. If you're panicking that you should be doing Zumba because it's the latest fad but you have no interest in sashaying to loud Latin music in a village hall, then *desist*.

3. **Tres.** It makes you feel good (see above).

4. **Cuatro.** It means you lose a sense of time. That feeling when two hours may have passed but it feels like twenty minutes.

5. **Cinq.** True plays means doing an activity with diminished self-consciousness. You are loving it so much that you don't care what you look like or whether you are any good at it. (Me dancing, now.)

6. **Seis. It has improvisational potential.** If the rules change a bit or you move on to a new game, then, without the desire for winning, you can be flexible and go with the flow.

7. **Sept. You want to keep doing it and will be sad it will end.** Which is why things like gym strength exercises or any adrenalin-spiking activities (like roller coasters) will never be play for me. I'm desperate for them to stop!

Play varies for us all. I won't be joining you for bridge and you may not want to come with me to *Mamma Mia!* I won't go jogging, but I will go on a mountain bike and screech 'wheeeeeeee' when going down even the smallest hill. I won't be doing a cryptic crossword (though I like some brain games), but I will be playing piano duets that I played when I was eleven. It's whatever you might remember your inner child would long to do. It's whatever you are able to do. It's whatever fits the above seven conditions as best as possible. Fly a kite? Cross-stitch? Whatever floats your boat. (And how delightful if floating your boat is your literal way to float your boat.) I still can't get enough of Lego. (Any Lego lovers who want to help me get a *Miranda* set of Lego, please write to me, or to Lego HQ. It's genuinely a life mission!) Play doesn't have to be silly. That's often where I veer. Play for you might be studying. Learning. Crying at the opera. Writing. Play for you might be helping out at the homeless shelter and chatting to people.

Those unique skills and ideas that make up who we are – it goes for play too. For example, as a highly sensitive person I know a music gig is not remotely play. It would thrill me but drain me. Put me in a quiet room listening to some Mozart and I'm at rest and play – particularly when I pretend to be the conductor, imagining I'm at the Royal Albert Hall . . .

Letting our imaginations fly is also a vital component to play. And why I was so glad my mind had started to dream again. In an open playful state, we are likely to be able to innovate and create in ways we would not otherwise. You never know, if you stop for a moment, give your imagination space to wander, you might just invent the next bestselling novel, or technological development, mode of transport, charitable initiative, medical cure, televisual blockbuster or garden pond. Somebody's got to. And that's what all great inventors ever did – they imagined. (P.S. You may need to put your phone down and dare to get bored for a moment to innovate in the ways you might be designed to. P.P.S. Scrolling is not play. Sorry!)

My route into the deepest, truest play is to find the things I'm not worried about being good at. That's my favourite definition. I love that play doesn't, as it were, have standards. That's a wholesome two fingers up to the productivity monster that I was beginning to see was emerging to be more and more the root cause of chronic stress and unhappiness in our culture. Play is never about a goal. The joy is in the doing, not the finishing.

A friend of mine and I, on learning all this, had a couple of Sundays doing a Crafts and Crisps Day. We bought a whole range of absurd crisps, some of which reminded us of our youth (Discos, anyone?), and some crafts that we knew we would be unskilled at. I chose a little ceramic, building-and-painting animal set. My elephant looked like a turd. And my duck looked like a . . . well, they all looked like turds because the mould split. I still painted them. Who says you can't polish a turd?!

Playing without any self-censorship is a revolutionary act of self-love and kindness.

Grateful For Gratitude

For me, the crucial by-product that came from play was gratitude. As I found ways to be playful, I had more to be grateful for; and the more I was grateful and felt the healing effects of that mindset, the more I wanted to find play and ensuing joy.

The research says that those with grateful minds are more naturally resilient. They're able to take their thoughts away from what they don't have, away from their difficult story, and on to what they do have and what they do love, right here, right now. As David Steindl-Rastl – an actual monk – writes, 'In daily life we must see that it is not happiness that makes us grateful, but gratefulness that makes us happy.' All hail the monkery-ness. I certainly feel more able to avoid the potholes now that I write twelve things I'm grateful for at the end of each day. A friend and I text each other every night with our twelve – such fun!

During any waiting for healing, waiting for news, waiting for situations to end, being grateful brings in trust and hope for the future, as well as an easier surrender for the now. It's not positive thinking; it's more powerful because what we are grateful for are concrete daily things right in front of us. We don't need to pine for a super-yacht; we can find the joy here. That is true resilience.

It's Completely Natural

The place that's always available to us, and free, is the great outdoors. Nature in all her splendour is there for us – the greatest adventure park and playground we could ever imagine. I would wager your greatest memories – moments of awe and wonder, challenges, excitement and therefore play – are within nature. No idea how to start playing? Let your mind wander to the childhood times you were discovering the outdoors.

When did you last build a sandcastle, MDRC? Can you feel yourself breathing out at the idea of bare feet on sand? I will never forget the screams of excitement when jumping in waves, whether aged nine or forty-nine (and, I hope, eighty-nine). The sea, such a gift – we can be on it, in it, splash, swim, surf, look at it, write about it, paint it. Our timeless, reliable friend, the sea. When did you last walk barefoot in grass? Intently listen to birdsong? Smell roses, literally? Cliché for good reason.

We have been duped, yet again, into thinking that there's no time to catch a falling leaf, watch a sunset, nap under the shade of a tree, dangle our feet in a river. How poorer we are for it. All the evidence shows people are healthier with access to green space, including behaviourally because of the calming effect. There was one study that indicated stress reduction within the brain when we put our hands in soil – showing why gardeners are among the healthiest professionals. And why I can be found with my hands dipped in my primula pot (not a euphemism) to feel the effect.

It's in our genes to need nature to tell us we are safe. For example, as you may know, MDRC, birdsong to our hunter-gatherer ancestors was an indication that there were no animals prowling, no immediate threat (the birds would go silent if there was danger). It's why we love birdsong so much. It literally makes us feel safe, and we can experience the physiological effect. As we sever our connection with nature more and more, the more stressed our bodies and minds can but become.

284

Author of *Wilding*, Isabella Tree (a little nod to the perfection of her surname), when writing about the rewilding of Knepp, tells us that rewilding is simply letting go and allowing nature to be the driver. If rewilding has been proved to bring back species never thought to be seen again, to let things flourish in the opposite way we thought would be better by controlling, the analogy is exact for our modern world. Like conventional conservation, our corporate capitalist world is about targets and control. It reminded me how I had treated *myself* as someone who should have goals to meet, a plan. I had been stuck on a worldly treadmill, a predicament of doing mode. Doing things I mainly wished I didn't have to do, dreaming of what I wanted to do. We are all too often suppressing ourselves and our nature. We are suppressing our instincts, our need to hibernate and rest, to just be, to play, to be still and quiet, to age, to express ourselves wildly and scruffily and not present 'perfectly'. It's a constant battle to go back to our wild selves. I love this from Isabella:

> As it grows old a tree sometimes lowers its branches to the ground for stability . . . like an old man using a walking stick. To the modern eye, this self-buttressing tendencey is considered a weakness and the walking stick – the lower branch – is generally removed . . . We deny the tree its ability to grow old, to gain character, to be itself.

We have a world in which to play, to enrich our every moment with awe and wonder, to grow old and be ourselves in. Let's get messy again. Let's let our hair look like we've gone through a hedge backwards – because we have. Let's get soil underneath our nails; let's let our mascara run down our faces in the rain; let's jump into a lake to swim, whatever we think of our bodies; let's let ourselves age disgracefully and look as exquisitely wrinkly as anything ageing in nature (I truly believe we look more beautiful the older and more natural we are); and let's support and encourage each other to do it all.

Walking

Without question, the times I've felt most well in various parts of my life have been in nature. When I pondered on why, for me, beyond the genetic evidence, I realized it was because it's always about movement. Even if I am still and just looking at it, nature will be moving, changing, dancing, swaying, rippling, twinkling.

Movement releases stuck energy and emotion, helps process thoughts, solves problems. When we walk, the nervous system can't remain in any fear-based fight, flight or freeze mode. The gentle movement indicates safety, and our body and mind become more optimistic, ready for challenges, feel more resilient. We instinctively say, 'Walk it off,' to someone tense or angry or stressed. It releases stored energy, it helps the immune system beat toxins and infections. There is such power in movement – even if we can just wiggle our toes and fingers.

We feel we want to conserve energy when fatigued, but actually the energy cells recover with movement, not without it. It can be very counterintuitive to go on a walk when you are lethargic, but if lethargy is often the repression of anger or grief rather than exhaustion, then movement mobilizes, releases and therefore re-energizes.

There's a book about walking called *Healing Walks for Hard Times* by Carolyn Scott Kortge. I recommend it generally, but particularly if you are recovering from burn-out, a significant operation or an illness. As Carolyn says, 'Walking sets the body's healing circulatory system in motion.' That said, understanding how much walking and movement to do is one of the hardest challenges of fatigue-based illnesses. Visualizing moving was so helpful before I could actually physically do it.

On which note, back to the amazing fact that the brain doesn't know the difference between the real and the imagined. There is extraordinary evidence on the healing power of imagining yourself doing activities as if you were well. Get this – in a study of people of similar age and build, those who lifted weights on an organized exercise programme gained 33 per cent more muscle tone, and – wait for it – those who only *imagined* lifting weights for the same number of weeks put on 22 per cent muscle tone. AMAZING. I visualized for my health in terms of physical movement. My body had become very weak and my brain saw exercise as a threat and caused huge fatigue crashes if I did the smallest amount. It was suggested I first visualize myself walking, with as much detail as I could, using senses of sight, sound and smell, and speaking out loud. I would imagine how strong and light I felt. What kind of terrain I was on. I cycled to the mountains and smelt the fresh air; I walked briskly by the sea, hearing the waves – I had some lovely adventures! I won an Olympic Gold in rowing once!

It was a better use of my imagination than any future cata-strophizing of my health condition. And it prepared my body. Believe it or not, I felt fitter. It became easier to walk without such fatigue crashes putting me back to bed for days. The body trusts the brain: it's practised this before. Just incredible.

It was such a brilliant discovery for the kind of illness I had because moving again is about incremental steps. My little 'rule', after visualizing, was to move within 50–70 per cent of capacity and stop before getting tired (I failed all the time!). I reckon it's a good rule for life. Capacity will natur-ally increase because the body can trust we are not going to push it.

A decade or so before I got very unwell, I met little Peggy and decided to bring her into my life. I genuinely think that the daily rhythm of walking Peggy stopped me getting sicker. (It was the time of TATT and having to just keep going.) I was in nature twice a day, experiencing weather that I hadn't for a long time living an office-based, urban life – it was crazy how I had avoided rain living in London and yet I blooming love getting wet and coming in to dry off. Rain is delicious. Smells delicious. Means stomping in puddles and mud (why do we stop doing that as adults?). Or a warm summer drizzle cooling you off. Being subjected to the weather because I had to walk the dog was a joyful privilege.

Now, big news incoming, MDRC: eleven months after Peggy died I took the leap to getting another puppy. It was a risk but it must have been instinctively the right time because my body adjusted to having to get up earlier and to do gentle walks around the garden. More than that, a puppy helped me start playing again. Play was the reason I was moving, not because of standards to get fit or get better. It was to take a gorgeous little animal outside to experience new things every day, which I then felt I was experiencing more mindfully anew. Dew on grass being licked and leapt around in (the puppy, not me – steady on), and I suddenly saw how beautiful a droplet of water on lush green grass is. Seeing her look up at a bird flying overhead with awe and amazement, and I did the same. I'm not suggesting everyone goes out and gets a puppy! But it was proof, to me, of what I had learnt. I was experiencing the physical and emotional lift of walking, nature and play. I don't believe, with the disease I had been dealt, I could have recovered without them.

Let me tell you more about said puppy. If you're not dying to know, then RUDE! Her full name, if you please: Dame Patience Pattercake Hart the Poochon of Portsmouth aka Patti aka a ball of light ginger fluff. She is a cross between a poodle and Bichon Frisé, hence 'poochon'. (Peggy was a Shih Tzu–Bichon Frisé cross – a 'Shitty Frisé' to my mind, so I seem to be covered in shit, if you pardon.)

Patti the Puppy heralded new beginnings. A ball of energetic, bumbling, tumbling joy that signalled my moving out from a time of waiting. Patti may have arrived in December, but she coincided with the light slowly dawning on my long hibernation.

A lot of people on first meeting Patti wondered if she was real, such was the teddy-bear-esque ball of fluff-ness, and everything she did was perfect auditioning for the cutest of all Disney films yet to be made. She befriended a toy kitten and carried it everywhere, making sure it experienced all the things she did. If she went to sleep, she'd get the kitten and press her nose against it like a kiss and then cuddle up with it. If she went outside, she would grab the kitten and place it, I jest you not, leaning up under a tree, as if giving it a view of her playing, with the little nose prod of affirmation: 'You just stay there and watch me run after the ball I am going to insist my tall owner throws for me.' She took baubles off the bottom of the Christmas tree and brought them to various relatives, usually at times when they needed some cheer. It was like living inside a cartoon.

Despite this absurd degree of cuteness, Patti's full name was Patience. And the true meaning of patience is anything but cute. The Latin word *pati* means 'to endure'. Patience is the ability to tolerate suffering without becoming annoyed or anxious. That's true warriorship right there. Surrender of the highest order. This fluff bundle was named to celebrate and honour my own time of unexpectedly lengthy endurance. Wondering – from the moment of lying collapsed looking at that sliding cat, through the long years of treatment, diagnosis, confusion and isolation – when or how or whether I may recover. The difficult memories and residue of endurance to get to full recovery needed the ridiculousness of a poochon to balance it out. (And it was joyful to be reunited with a dog to stroke – a perfect example of my brain receiving natural neurotransmitters.)

If ever you bump into us, feel free to tell us if you're in a time of darkness – we might just be on for a cuppa, or at the very least a cuddle and a lick. Patti would do the licking, to be clear. My love for you reading my little story does not extend to any kind of licking. Let's move on, it's getting weird . . .

Pottery

A good and important friend is one to whom you can say, with no context, 'We should go and find a pottery class, shouldn't we?' and they respond, 'Most definitely,' and you just know that one of you will be sending a link and it will be happening asap.

When life first started opening up for me again, and I found myself with pleasure-seeking playful options of these kinds, it was an extraordinary moment. Talk about grateful. I said to myself, 'Why on earth haven't I done a pottery class before? I love the idea of pottery.' I felt wistful. It brought it home how my life had left less and less room just for pleasure, when it's part of my very essence. Off we pottered!

We were given a smock, shown to our wheels, refrained from immediately going into the *Ghost* pose (though the desire was strong), and the teacher gave us a little demonstration of a basic pot.

As an aside: I've decided that adults need to wear smocks or big shirts worn back to front more. We did that in primary school. When did the smock-wearing stop?! I feel sure that those in aprons and smocks who make a mess are the happiest of people.

I couldn't wait to get my hands on that clay and make a mess. I couldn't wait to be really bad at something and not care. I couldn't wait to play.

I was having some beginner's luck with my pot. Pot luck – thank you! My friend was rather envious – hers looked like a droopy mushroom (and that's being kind). After I removed my first one, rather pleased with myself, I started with a fresh lump of clay, and a fresh degree of enthusiasm. This time I decided I wanted to make the pot shorter and wider. I was aiming for more of a dog bowl for Patti (what the hell did I know!). I was concentrated and steady and this lovely wide bowl emerged. My friend said, 'Wow, that's crazy, how did you do that?' The teacher was impressed but warned, 'Careful the walls don't become too thin,' suggesting I leave it there. But I didn't want to leave it there. I wanted to make it better. I was on a winning streak pottery-wise and so I pushed it to its limit, this little dog bowl of mine. Sure enough, the walls became too thin, crumbled and collapsed inwards. Deceased pot. It looked like an Art Deco ashtray.

I said to my friend – who not only knows me well but happens to be a therapist – how interesting that I pushed that pot to its max, not stopping when it and others were telling me to; let's not ignore the fact that I've been known to do that to myself. I sat for a moment looking at my dog-bowl-turned-ashtray-turned-floppy-mess-turd-of-clay, and acknowledged this playful experience had turned into a way to make a promise to myself. A promise that when I was out in the world again, I would stop when my body (or the clay, if I was to become a potter) told me to. That I would understand my limits and know that accepting them showed strength and courage and was just darn sensible. I was getting out and about more with a slow degree of healing, and please know the only thing I did was discover these treasures (I didn't have any special pill or potion), but I was always going to have to practise them, and pace myself. Which, joyfully, would always mean the need to play. Let's never forget, MDRC, it's play that recharges and restores.

My hunch that following joy breeds more joy was affirmed when The Boy, having heard the above potting story, got me a present of a pottery class for us both – massive brownie points. I was falling for Patti, and daring to hope maybe I wouldn't just have a dog husband this time, but I kept focusing on my recovery. *Pace yourself, Miranda!* And that was indeed the next treasure.

P.S. I Got Better With Play

I don't think many people, if they'd come into my bedroom to see a very weak, ashen-faced me, would say, 'Tell you what you need, dear – a game of Jenga?' or, 'Up you get, let's bop, I'll pop on some ABBA.' It can seem a counterintuitive choice to focus on joy, but that still-small voice that whispered to me that morning was spot on. The harder it feels to play, the more it's worth summoning the courage to do just that.

I think this was the most practical treasure for my healing. Looking towards joy is the most important part of rewiring the stress response. Let me quickly remind you of that concept. I'm so flipping excited that it's slowly filtering down from neuroscientists' studies over the last four or five decades to GP

293

clinics and becoming the understood universal answer in the healing of many chronic illnesses, in particular ME/CFS, fibromyalgia, food and chemical sensitivities, and now long Covid. But many are yet to know or understand it so if there's one thing I'm going to be evangelical about, it's this. I feel forever grateful I scientifically know that the brain is the home for the immune, hormonal and nervous systems. The key systems we need to fight disease. When that brain becomes lower in energy, it is not balanced well enough to send healthy messages to the immune system to order itself, to flush out the toxins and viruses. It gets stuck on high alert, as it does when we are first infected, and continues to pour adrenalin and fighting chemicals into our body as part of the survival mechanism. And that, along with all the existing activated diseases, keeps us sick. If we start to send signals to the brain consistently (it takes a few months or more – years in my case) that we are safe, if the brain notices we are actually 'playing', it lights up, and the immune system will feel safe and go, 'Oh, hold fire, the main threat is over, we're okay, we can stop giving her so many symptoms now to force her to rest, stand down.' The immune system reorders, the nervous system goes back to a healing state, the hormonal system regulates again and many symptoms and conditions simply ebb away. IT'S AMAZING, MDRC. It tells you that joy and play are genuine ways to keep healthy, fight disease and prolong your life. And, I remembered from Treasure Four (Thoughts), the way to move away from negative thoughts is to pivot to an intentional joyful distraction, so to have play at our fingertips can but help our brain grow healthier thought trees.

This treasure cemented a decision I was coming to. After much time, energy and money spent on complicated medical protocols after diagnosis with little effect, I decided to only do the brain rewiring to recover. I was more disciplined to rewire away from my negative thought loops about my health, stopped mitigating against or trying to solve symptoms, and stopped trying to work out whether what I was doing was helping me get better or not. All those things were causing stress. Instead, I acted as best I could within the limitations I had. I slowly did things for joy. Very gently, one step at a time. I fake-smiled (and sometimes, if I dared, 'ho, ho, ho-ed'!), I sat up, I started to make gratitude lists. I visualized wellness. It was hard to start with, until it truly wasn't. Until I went from being bed-bound to sitting upright to do Lego. Until I slowly felt less poisoned and less toxic, until I felt more hope. Until I could go for a gentle walk. Surrendering became easier because my life wasn't just about being ill; it was about the things I now did every day that I wanted to do *despite* my illness.

I wasn't just naming the good; I was adding in, 'How good can I let this moment be?' (I do this often now regardless.) Shall I open the window and feel the breeze on my face? Shall I listen to some music? How can I transport my mind to deviate from the story I have been stuck in and stop flapping in agitation like that butterfly against my bedroom window? I could persevere, even when the acts felt small, because I knew that by staying with a nice, safe experience, I was creating lasting change on a cellular level. I was closer to coming home to that true core identity that brought health. And now part of that identity is the next value to join the party, the glaringly obvious watchword for this treasure: joy. Oh, how joyful to discover that!

Treasure Eight

Pacing and Presence

TREASURES PICKED UP: Intentional, calm, simplicity, habitual, celebratory, restful, learning how you uniquely tick, going step-by-step and one day at a time

PATTERNS SMASHED: Busyness, rushing, numbed out, asleep to bad habits, changing who you are to 'be normal', craving better than the now

WATCHWORD: Gentleness

SOUNDTRACK: 'Perfect Moment' by Martine McCutcheon

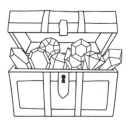

Pacing and Presence

Intentional Pottering

One of my favourite pastimes is pottering. I don't mean walking; in fact, a potter does not get close to resembling a walking stride. There's no rushing involved, but a very slow, intentional and relaxing amble. A shuffle of an Italian nonagenarian if you will.

My twenty-something assistant just asked me, 'What are you writing about?'

'Intentional pottering.'

An intriguing reply came back: 'Oh wow, do people do it unintentionally?'

'I think so, yes,' I answered. 'People either waste time not really knowing they're doing it; some, I think, fear it, think it's somehow wrong or "old"; some have never even considered it . . .'

'People think it's wrong? That's so weird to me.' This was getting more intriguing.

'Well, it's quite weird to me that you are giving it such thought. It feels quite a middle-aged consideration . . .'

She seemed slightly offended. 'I might be young and have a lot to learn but I have heard of and even done some pottery.'

'Pottery or pottering?' I asked, seeing where it may have gone wrong.

'What? What's pottering?' The order of things was restored.

Suffice to say, twenty-two-year-olds probably don't necessarily know what I mean by 'intentional pottering'. And please don't think I mean intentional pottery. I imagine all potters are very intentional otherwise there'd be carnage with clay flying left, right and centre in any given pottery class – 'Marjorie, can you be more intentional, please? The handle of your jug whacked me in the face.' All sorts of amusing images are coming to mind . . . though I admit I did cause minor carnage when I went to my pottery class. I opened the door to the warehouse space, not noticing there was a step down, and stumbled in loudly, using a shelf of newly glazed pots to steady myself. The other potters gasped as the pots wobbled, and then they all turned to me. I chose to wave heartily with a jaunty, public school, 'Hello, potting peeps!' I was also unable to refrain from making fake noses for myself and my friend to pot with.

Let's get back to my pottering pastime. My favourite thing about it being how utterly and gloriously gentle it feels. To move deliberately in the opposite pace to the frantic world, to have time to breathe and absorb all around. Time to look up. In fact, my watchword for this treasure is . . . gentleness. Oh, the joy of gentleness.

We live in a world that seemingly lacks gentleness. From hooting traffic jams to packed, stampeding commutes (still longing for the statutory gallop on a commute), to the sound of keyboards, ringtones, car alarms, sirens – it's all so jumpy, nothing soft about it. But within our abrasive, concrete institutions there will be stunning moments of gentleness we rarely see. A teacher whispering a word of encouragement. A nurse holding a hand and taking a moment to smile and breathe with a patient. A colleague helping another with their paper jam (there's nothing gentle about a massive photocopier, let alone when it jams . . .). Perhaps if we can create more moments of gentleness within this frantic world, we may help slow it – and ourselves – down to a more natural pace. A gentle revolution of gentleness.

It might seem futile and silly to say that some intentional pottering is a good way to start, but in all my experiments of slowing down, it's the one that has made the biggest difference. And there's even a scientific reason for pottering, MDRC. If we rush, we send signals to our brain that we might be under threat; the nervous system does its thing and fires up in anticipation, causing a spike in cortisol and adrenalin. Noticing how shallow my breathing became when rushing was fascinating, too. Shallow breathing also tells our brain we are under threat. Slowing down calms our body as the brain thinks, 'Oh, we are moving more slowly, right, we are safe now, stand down.' It was another key to reducing my chronic stress response. Things were continuing to feel lighter.

301

There are still only twenty-four hours in each day, but on the days I go slower it truly feels like I have created more hours. Life feels simpler – gentler. Slowing down also helps me be more intentional about the activities and tasks I choose to do in the day, how I go about them and for how long. The 'ists' were right – slowing down is the way to make oneself more present, which therefore allows one to make better choices.

I was heartened, yet again, by how the treasures were revealing themselves to be gentle. (Of course true ways for our holistic health would be kind and gentle.) At the start of my experience, options for well-being didn't feel doable, accessible or simple to add into my every day. Often, they felt another thing to strive for. But not the treasures. They were nothing but kindly gifts, despite the depth of insight underpinning them.

If simply slowing down is a gentle prescription to help our brain and body function optimally, I highly recommend experimenting with pottering – slow your walking pace getting from A to B, do daily household tasks more slowly, pause and take three deep breaths before you check your emails. It all makes a difference.

A great tip for women, particularly those with a larger breasticle, is to practise intentional pottering by not wearing a bra! It slows down my walk naturally, for without a bra any movement looks like I'm smuggling ferrets under my armpits . . . Plus, isn't it freeing to be braless for a moment? I feel without care the instant I remove my bra. I might feel the weight of the breast, but the weight of life is removed! You are oh so very welcome for the images I have just conjured for you, MDRC – my absolute pleasure.

P.S. We could start a pottering club and confound the world with our joyful, slow amble, Miranda's amble – a Miramble, if you will (pleased with that).

Hot, Hot, Hot

Another time I naturally excel at pacing myself and moving calmly and mindfully is when I am hot. When it gets over about twenty-seven degrees, I don't cope very well. I become a limp yet angry husk. It's quite the combo. Let's just say I am not my best self in the heat. I care very little for anything or anyone in my hot grumpiness except ice and ice cream. I've been known to stand in my bra and pants in the garden and shout, 'Please to hose me down forthwith as a matter of urgency!' (More imagery for you that's my pleasure to bestow.) I care not what the neighbours may think, I simply cannot cope a moment longer in my swollen, hot body.

The upside on very hot days of sweating profusely is that I'm forced to move extremely leisurely and I become exceptionally good at this treasure. Despite the hot, hot anger caused by my hot, hot hotness, I am calmed. If taking some breaths and moving more slowly can chill an angry, hot woman ... why would I move any other way during a day with an acceptable temperature?

The Emergency Walk

In my sitcom there was a scene in which 'Miranda' and her best friend Stevie did what they called their emergency walk. They were on an urgent mission and they decided to get their alert, fast-paced, military walk on. They saluted to each other and stormed off comedically emergency-walk style-y. This came from a real-life event when my sister and I were travelling in South Africa. We got a flat tyre on our hire car, and my sister went into a complete tailspin, her mind convincing her that we were about to be kidnapped. The reality was we were in a safe, suburban restaurant car park. But off she went, storming like a deranged army colonel, so fast that I had to jog after her to ask her where she was going. She had no idea, she just panicked and her body took her to an 'emergency walk'.

Sometimes, when she gets in after the school run at the pace of a hurricane and begins furiously chopping carrots, I suggest that the carrots would only get chopped approximately 3.7 seconds slower if she'd calm down. The house isn't on fire, let's get off emergency status. It doesn't always go down well saying that to a busy mother (the most noblest of creatures) when everyone in the house is demanding something of her. But the point stands.

The problem, as ever, comes when these kinds of less-than-helpful behaviours become more regular. When the sense that to get something done, to tick off the to-do list, to get the children to school, to get to work on time, even to complete exercise or leisure time, means bringing out the 'emergency walk'. When we end up doing life as if the ground is moving too fast for us and we fear we will never get things done.

When I first became aware of this, I was both alarmed and amused at how fast my thinking and physical pace often were. Even getting out of bed – it was like someone had fired a starting gun. Quick: get my clothes on – as if someone was timing me – rush down to the kettle, open my laptop with fear of what might have popped into my inbox overnight. On lunch breaks my thoughts were often on what the afternoon held, and I would wolf my food down, perceiving it as an irritant in the way of what I next had to do. Now I am aware of pacing and presence, if I notice I'm in emergency mode, I take a breath and move slower. Now, I always try to savour the gift of a meal. Now, I take a moment on first waking to smile, be grateful for a new day and take three long, deep breaths.

We have caught the frantic pace of our modern world, and it's just not good for us, MDRC. If I ever get back to work in an office or on a television project, I will boldly make room in my diary for stillness. It's those moments within a day where the real excitement, gentleness, unexpectedness and curiosity will be. And more to the point, I will be operating from rest, at a pace that doesn't put unnecessary pressure on my body, and therefore I will be more productive. (Plus, if I can do that, then I won't have to whip my bra off in an office to slow myself . . .)

What Is Rest?

I've been thoroughly enjoying regaling you with images of me braless, being hosed down on a hot day or trying to behave in a pottery class, but I shall buckle up for a moment, for I want to share something I found super interesting and important about rest.

It is, of course, essential for us humans to rest. What I found so useful, which I excitedly share with you now, MDRC, in case you didn't know, is that there are seven types of rest – physical, mental, spiritual, sensory, creative, emotional and social. They speak to all of our key needs.

Physical rest is the most obvious – a good night's sleep, a nap or a longer holiday (if we should be so lucky). Or just being horizontal from time to time where we can – I'll lie down wherever (bed shop, anyone?). Learning the other types of rest, I found, took the pressure off any lack of physical rest at times. I know I am not alone in the sometimes ludicrous worry of 'I must get eight hours' sleep' and if I wake up and it's been seven hours and forty-six minutes, 'Oh God, the day's RUINED!' If we're able to create time in the day or week for the other types of rest, our sleep will likely improve as the body will generally be more relaxed.

Mental rest is simply time without a task. It might be finding a mindfulness routine that works for you, or simply looking away from screens. For me, it's usually staring into the distance or up at the sky. Watching a passing cloud. Giving my mind a quick break.

Emotional rest might mean finding moments to feel how we feel, letting emotions move through us, sharing an experience – I know, for instance, that if I don't have a little cry every few days, then I am probably keeping things in.

That's just me – I need a regular weep, joyful or otherwise.

Creative rest helps me if I've been looking at the potholes for too long. On realizing I have become weighed down by problems or issues, I know I need to hop to some joy and play.

I love that the list of rest types includes sensory because we truly live in sensory overload. The biggest culprits, of course, are our beloved and dreaded smartphones. Putting our phones down is SO hard. But the 'ists' tell us that the general anxiety increase so many of us experience around phone usage is usually because of exhausting overstimulation, rather than the content that's necessarily absorbed. Looking down in a slumped posture, with glaring light, darting images, noise and speed-reading content can't help but keep the brain frenzied and wired. Without sensory rest, we can't control the overwhelm. If in doubt, look up. Give your neck and shoulders a rest. There are restful senses to follow too, like putting our hands in soil if you remember (not always easy in an office – though perhaps we should have pots of soil around for said dipping).

Spiritual rest is harder to pin down, as it will vary for all. My go-to is nature, finding the awe and believing there's something bigger that is loving and for me. To feel held by. That immediately settles me in frantic moments.

And finally, social rest. Well, I can only speak as an introvert whose way to socially recharge is to have a meal in a darkened room on my own. I know for you extroverts, you need to recharge with a big night out or some long chats. (Weirdos – joke!)

There is an adage that I've never forgotten because of my health history, and since reading it I try to have moments of each type of rest every day (however small): 'If you listen to your body when it whispers, you won't have to hear it scream.' And there it is: our bodies need rest to reduce inflammation, to detox from processed foods, environmental factors, stress, other people, viruses and infections, fear and worry. You may want to shout at me, as I used to shout at the 'ists': 'Well, Miranda, it all sounds lovely, but my life is in a pickle and I feel rubbish, and pottering, or doing a hobby, or looking at the sky, let alone shoving my hands in soil, sounds silly and annoying or not possible. I'm so tired I just want to cry.' Oh, my lovely dearest of reader chums, I so hear you. I think that all any one of us can do is look for whatever the next loving action might be.

Here's a little listicle of little things that might help a little. I found it crazy hard when I started to move away from the tasks I wanted to get done and find times to do things like this, but the difference really was palpable.

- ◈ Potter – obviously the first one.
- ◈ Stretch – doesn't have to mean donning Lycra and doing a session on a gym mat, I just mean putting arms above head at your desk to try and get a little stretch and yawn (if a yawn naturally comes, it means you are detoxing stress – very satisfying).
- ◈ Regularly stop to drop shoulders – mine are often around my ears when at my desk.
- ◈ Set a timer for five minutes to look away from all screens. Maybe close your eyes and notice where your body hurts and needs to relax.

- ◈ Listen to a song – lots of research shows the healing power of instrumental music in particular.
- ◈ Splash your face with cold water and/or sip ice-cold water – this has a calming effect and doesn't require the whole extreme ice bath thing that doesn't suit many.
- ◈ Look at nature or videos of nature, or comedic animal videos – the best reason the internet was invented, in my opinion.
- ◈ Smile or fake-smile – I often type with a fake smile and get less frantic when I do; it sometimes makes me feel weird to start with but I don't care! The body doesn't know the difference, so you might as well help it along.
- ◈ Eat less sugar – I went on quite the snack journey to discover some that were actually healthy and not hideously disgusting.
- ◈ Have some salt or electrolytes or a big glass of water.
- ◈ Take omega-3 and vitamin D.
- ◈ Name five things you are grateful for.
- ◈ Do a random act of kindness.
- ◈ Become aware of any top ten thought tunes that might be scaring you, and remember they are not the truth. Do the five questions on a piece of paper to dismantle them.
- ◈ Ask for help – got to keep practising that one, MDRC.
- ◈ Ask for a hug – where appropriate; might be best to wait until after the job interview . . .
- ◈ And there's always galloping, if you are able!

Once I started to practise rest I soon realized that my successful attempts had something in common – they were each bringing me more into the present moment. I had not been in the present much, it turned out. You can't be, if you are a rusher and a planner and a doer to the exclusion of rest. And it's often hard, when sick, because you simply don't want to be present. I was inspired by the story of Vidyamala Burch, a woman who has lived with severe pain from a number of accidents and is, in the main, wheelchair-bound. She became a mindfulness expert after an epiphany. The only way, she realized, that she would be able to cope with her agony was to know that she only had to get through the present moment. Not even the whole day, just the present moment . . .

> *I saw that the present moment is manageable, and I felt the confidence this knowledge brought. Fear drained out of me and I relaxed. I realized that much of my torment had grown out of fear of the future – the future moments of pain that I imagined stretching on forever – rather than what I was actually experiencing in the present moment. I was 'pre-feeling' my future pain and worry, as well as having to cope with the present-moment suffering. I was needlessly multi-plying my pain.*

So thought-provoking, MDRC. I acknowledged how much I had been pre-feeling and pre-thinking events, which can *only* be scary. (As ever, judging ourselves with where we are at can be as painful as the painful situation we are experiencing.)

Busy, Busy, Busy

When I get asked to do anything, the first line of the email or text will invariably be, 'I know you must be sooo busy but . . .'

or, 'I know you are such a busy woman but . . .' as if busyness is a crown, a badge of honour. Being frantically, and often detrimentally, busy is another unhelpful pattern many of us have come to believe means fulfilment or self-worth. But surely it's a symptom of the success trap and doesn't honour our 'why'?

Being productive, doing what needs to get done, nurturing our skills are all brilliant and necessary things – I am often at my happiest at work – but it's the pace, MDRC. The way we do things, the expectation, the striving, the working conditions. The long hours. The cry of 'there just isn't enough time'. Lots of 'I don't have the choice'. I remembered often wishing time would stop still for a month or two so I could catch my breath and have a rest. There seems to be a lack of trust in employers – as if everyone has become scared to be human, with needs. People seem scared to have limits within the workplace. Linked, I suppose, to being scared to be vulnerable.

Did you know that since 2019, the World Health Organization has identified burn-out as a serious occupational phenomenon, defining it as 'a syndrome conceptualized as resulting from chronic workplace stress that has not been successfully managed'. Sobering. We now live in a world whose health organization has had to define a syndrome based on how poorly we can treat ourselves and each other. How some companies (not all and not all knowingly) are rinsing their employees' life forces under their noses. I have had parents tell me the same too – that there is a lot of burn-out with expectations around parenting.

There was a time I might have shied away from anything resembling a passionate ramble. Not now. Here I am in all my blazing glory! And my rally cry is this: we need a gentle revolution of gentleness to create a world in which people can follow their ambitions, creativity and working ideas without pushing themselves to the limit. Where we understand and acknowledge that productivity increases with rest (and play), as do our health and happiness, therefore we need a world in which time for rest and recharging is incorporated and celebrated. It's my Pottering Crusade!

I felt encouraged my suspicions were right but also a little sickened when I read a *Harvard Business Review* article by Charlotte Lieberman, in which she wrote:

> ... *we continue to glamorize being overworked, busy, and stressed ... This might explain why counting our steps and recording our exhales are satisfying ways to measure the success of our self-care routine once we leave the office. But in this context, our high anxiety becomes just another thing to 'work on'.*

Another sobering moment as I realized many are approaching wellness with the same oppressive energy as they might do their careers. I had another celebratory moment of the treasures being my new and gentle way.

I can't speak for you, MDRC, but I'd been known back in the day to do steps on the spot in the kitchen when tired, just to hear my Fitbit ping to 10,000 steps. RIDICULOUS! It doesn't work to be in a frantic state to help our franticness. It's not kind or loving. If we are more scared about our health because of all the articles we are reading and the exercise fads we can't keep up with, and we're more scared about our sleeping because an app says our REM cycle is out of whack, and we're scared to indulge in a nice piece of cake because of the fat and sugar content, then I suggest (hark me getting impassioned again) that that anxiety is far worse than savouring a delicious slice of Victoria sponge. Look at people who are in their seventies, eighties and nineties – many of them have never eaten goji berries or heard of Reformer Pilates. They have a simpler way of living, eating in moderation, being in face-to-face connection and going about at a more natural pace. Because they grew up at a time pre-'frantic'.

There is nothing virtuous about torturing ourselves. It's so unnervingly easy to get into the cycle of avoiding tiredness by staying busy and then crashing. Recharging just enough to go back to a fast pace to get things done, and then crashing again. Back to the boom-and-bust cycle that can cause chronic fatigue. Slowing down is vital for getting out of these cycles of busyness and listening to what type of rest our mind and body need.

The cycle of busyness makes me think of the saying that the definition of insanity is doing the same thing over and over again and hoping for a different outcome. (I suppose that's what I was doing when I kept pushing myself, before I understood surrender.) Don't rush and busy yourself to impress. It's the least impressive thing to do. I know I'm not playing the game any more. I will be found pottering slowly without a bra at any given opportunity. (I will not gallop without a bra – the world isn't ready for that . . . yet . . .)

'How You Do One Thing Is How You Do Everything'

I'm not sure we know who coined the phrase 'How you do one thing is how you do everything', but I think it is completely brilliant. It showed me the problem is about the *way* we do things, not necessarily *what* we are doing.

It reminded me of the time I was mulling about putting the emergency walk into my comedy when I found myself doing it in a shopping mall. I'm not a fan of shopping at the best of times, but I had to get something, and I became irritated-slash-full-on-furious because I couldn't understand the massive mall map on the annoyingly slow touch screen thingy! Out came the emergency walk as I mumbled, 'Fine, I will just march through the stupid mall and find the stupid shop myself then if the stupid map is that stupidly confusing.' I heard a wise whisper: *How you do one thing is how you do everything, Miranda.* Did I want to be an irritable, angry marcher in all things I do? No, I wished to be a serene lady wafting elegantly through life patiently, playfully, peacefully and powerfully. If I could practise this in a shopping mall, then I was more likely to be this person on the days that needed the best of me. I started doing a walk that resembled as much of an 'elegant waft' as I could muster. And there it was: immediately on slowing my pace, I had time to enjoy what was around me, I smiled at another, I felt instantly a nicer person! The task was still going to get done, but this time with values and health intact.

It's not what you do, it's the state you are in when you do it.

314

I also, in that moment, treated myself better. And here is the pinnacle of my passionate ramble (or Miramble) – we are only ever going to want to improve something we think is worth improving. Yup, it keeps coming back to that, MDRC. When we steadfastly believe that our inherent identity is one of value, we stop perceiving ourselves as something to fix. Instead, we honour the way we function best. We then feel safe to go at our own pace, and we're able to be present for all the good we'd miss by running.

Don't run from yourself, MDRC, you're a glorious elephant!

The Still, Small Voice

As I brought more stillness and presence into my life, I was reacquainted with a part of me that had been all too often silenced in the busyness of my past. My still, small voice within. The opposite of the inner critic. The voice that knows I have nothing to prove and wants only to give me a gift of a thought, a moment of fun, a connection, an exciting idea to develop. A memory that brings healing laughs and tears. The nudging voice reminding me of a forgotten but long-held passion. The gentle prod that tickles my conscience and tells me it's time to make amends. The loving reminder to take some rest.

Some may call it gut instinct, others God, or creativity, or love, or spirit. To me it's the voice that somehow I know to be true. It's the kindest, gentlest voice from beyond the world's noise. The one that told me to lie in the sun that May day and let it feel like an IV of love. It was the creative instinct that told me, way back when, to pitch a ridiculous-sounding show to the BBC about a woman who runs a joke shop and looks to camera (when producers were advising me that was an unlikely sell). It's the voice that told me I needed little Peggy, even though it didn't make practical sense as a single, busy thirty-something in a London flat. It was the one that said ditch the protocols and trust the 'ists' and the treasures. It was the one that said just write out your poem ideas, even though you know nothing about poetry.

Because I had been living without the presence in the moment that would enable me to hear my guiding inner voice, it was like I had sleepwalked through a lot of my life. Been on autopilot. Almost as if choices had been made for me, not by me. I wish I had been a little surer of my instincts in my earlier decades, and listened to that voice for better choices. I would often seek other people's advice, wanting someone to decide things for me. Now I often go with the simple wisdom of: 'Does it feel life-giving or life-draining? Joyful or worrying?' I remind myself not to put myself under pressure to get it 'right'. There's not always going to be a clear right path to go down exactly. But, with value-based living at the fore, I finally had a solid platform from which to make decisions.

Recently, I was able to listen to my instincts about having Patti the Poochon from Portsmouth and The Boy from Bristol in my life! I was sure it was right to invest in these two lovely relationships. But that didn't mean they were without fear or trepidation. There were many tearful nights, during the early pooing and peeing puppy stage, wondering what I had done. And being attracted to someone can come with a myriad of insecurities. But because both decisions came from that still, small voice within, I had the confidence to go ahead, and the gumption to ignore any inner criticism/shouts to the opposite.

The Rogue Whippet

I was granted such a hilarious, joyful moment by being more present recently, MDRC. I took Patti around the block (she also loves a good potter), and a sweet white whippet without a lead came bounding up to us in the street. I thought she belonged to a woman getting into a nearby car, so I let Patti play and have a moment with the whippet. But then said woman closed her car door and drove off. I looked around and there was no one in the street. I had a rogue whippet on my hands. Interesting! I was having a break from writing an article I needed to get done that day, and there was a fleeting thought from the past of, *This is annoying, I don't have time to deal with a stray dog, I want to finish my writing.* But I let it fly off so that I could enjoy the adventure of this moment. The obvious next step with my new whippet friend was to call the number on her tag. I dialled and the number was not recognized. Interesting! I decided the next step was to pick Patti up and put the whippet on my lead. I did so and started walking back. And then I got giggly because I thought, *Well, hang on, now what? I seem to own a whippet now and I'm taking her home. Is this my new life?!* The whippet suddenly dived down to a basement flat. She must have known it. I went down to knock on the door, but it was unlocked and slightly ajar. I did the classic 'Helloooooooo' in the doorway but heard nothing. There was another dog in there – a large greyhound. It made sense that this was probably the

317

whippet's home. I placed her in there, put Patti back on her lead and went on my merry way. Then I started giggling again. What if the sweet white whippet didn't live there, and someone came home to randomly find a new dog in their sitting room?! And what if the bigger greyhound started fighting her or something and there was a bloodbath? And then – oh my God, maybe the whippet does belong there, but the owner is passed out or dead in their flat and I should have gone in further to check?! Oh yes, I was fully present to all scenarios with this unexpected twist in my day. I went home and decided to write a note to say if it wasn't their dog, then this was my number if they needed help.

As I approached the flat (again, the briefest moment of irritation at my time slipping by when I wanted to be writing, quickly ignored for the excitement of it all), I realized I should probably also look for a dead body. I did another 'Helll-loooooooo' on opening the door and crept further in. (Why do we think more Os make us sound friendlier? It's surely weirder!) Luckily no dead body, but a man on his patio doing some gardening. I knocked on the closed French windows; he stared, shocked, and didn't move. I was giggling again, because of course he didn't realize his front door was open. I was by now holding the whippet; I opened the French window and said, 'Sorry to disturb you, but is this your dog?' 'Yes,' he said, bemused. By this point I was giggling even more – to him it just looked like a random stranger had broken into his flat to ask if his dog was his dog!! As I explained, he looked mostly relieved but still a bit shaky. He said, 'I thought someone was playing a prank because you are my favourite person on television.' (A man of exceptionally good taste.) The whole thing was completely ridiculous. I ended our exchange with, 'I'm just glad you are not dead,' which of course made no sense to him as he didn't know I had perhaps thought he was, and I laughed the whole way home, beyond excited to tell the whole thing to The Boy, who I was seeing later that night.

I was so glad my past pattern of rushing to get a task done had been smashed so as to have enjoyed the minutiae of this silly, mini escapade. I love being in connection and in the present. I *love* being awake to all aspects of my life. Finally. The light, the dark, the sublime, the ridiculous. I can even have symptoms I am able to ignore and they usually lift as a result. Simply, I am happy to be here.

The Boy

In part, I had The Boy to thank for learning to be present. A year or so before getting to whippet-level-brush-the-thoughts-away presence, he had suggested we go on a trip away together. I was incredibly excited to be able to say yes. It was my first ever trip beyond the small confines of home and family – this was pre sinking mud, Knepp, etc. We were headed to Dorset, in case you desire to know, MDRC. The landscape seemed so surreally beautiful and dramatic. The only other time I had seen scenery like it in recent years was in films. I was stepping out on to nature's film set (ooh, that's a bit naff, but I like it). Yet among the excitement, old patterns were rearing. As they do. I went into busy planning mode to make sure I made the trip as 'successful' as possible. 'I want to walk to Durdle Door, kayak at Lulworth Cove, see Lulworth Castle, go to two RSPB sites and visit three restaurants.' The Boy pointed out that I was still recovering from fatigue and needed to pace myself. Hello, old pattern of wanting to 'nail it', 'do it well or not at all', 'do it right'. What does 'do it right' even mean? Talk about taking the joy out of life.

In the moment, I got a little gloomy. I so longed to have a level of health and energy that meant I could walk as long and as far as I liked, that meant I could get in a car and go on trips without concern. The Boy was inspired: 'What's to say that staying in one place, with one view, and exploring one small area is any less adventurous and successful than seeing all the so-called "top spots"?' So that's what we did.

It's a holiday I will never forget. I have had the luxury of going to many top holiday destinations in my time, but this was better than all of those. We were both being intentionally present, which meant being more grateful and more joyful, and – most thrillingly (which you can't buy at any exclusive hotel) – my mind stopped racing. I learnt a host of bird names and their songs. I will never forget a wimbrel, and its melodic tune, until the day I die. I saw a kingfisher for the first time and won't forget that flash of shimmering blue underbelly. I never thought I would be a person who could stare at the intricacies of an oak tree for lengths of time, feeling genuinely awed and captivated. Rushing means we miss that the world can be a benevolent place. It is there for our safety, our adventure, our wonder, our fun. When you experience its microcosmic gentle beauty, you can see that. The gift of The Boy saying let's just stay in this one spot, in this garden, with these views, and be. My peaceful mindset allowed my body to recharge. If, instead, I'd emergency-walked all over the local castles on day one, I would have crashed.

I acknowledged tearily that I had been too fearful to be present in my life before now. Fearful of physical symptoms, of restriction, that my future would never be all I longed for.

Hark at this spot of spirituality. A great theologian, Tim Keller, recently admitted in an article in *The Atlantic* that he and his wife, living with a new perspective since his terminal cancer diagnosis:

> ... have discovered that the less we attempt to make this world into a heaven, the more we are able to enjoy it. No longer are we burdening it with demands impossible for it to fulfil. We have found that the simplest things—from sun on the water and flowers in the vase to our own embraces, sex, and conversation—bring more joy than ever. This has taken us by surprise.

I was so grateful for their honesty. Despite trying to live by the values of their faith, they were still stuck in busy, busy, busy – until they saw that what was in front of them was what they wanted to savour.

I could agree. The cave was finally getting lighter.

If You Never Get To Santorini, That's Okay

I spent many years as a slave to idealism, and being present in one place on that Dorset trip freed me. My lofty goals, my planning, my yearnings for excitement and adventure had all seemed like the right answer. The best way I could live and enjoy my life. But I often suffered from disappointment because many desires were never satisfied – or I didn't see the present moment as good enough. As another mindfulness expert, Dr Dan Siegel, says, 'Presence makes you happy, happiness doesn't make you happy.'

The 'perfect' holiday I'd idealized was Grecian island hopping. What was I hoping that hopping around Greek islands would produce in me? How was I expecting I would come back differently?

During my illness, my life had been restricted. I battled the frustration that this produced. Now, though, I could see that all I wanted was to not want. To be satisfied with whatever life threw at me, whether that was a glorious beach cove on Santorini or a sickbed. For I was now of the belief that there is always something loving and nourishing in every present moment.

For so many of us, our desires are simply not possible. I felt (and still feel) that all that mattered were the values I was learning from the cave. Perhaps, I don't know, uncovering these treasures was going to be my most important adventure? The adventure to that wild self.

But I do know that if I never get to Santorini, that's totally okay!

What Have You Done Today To Make You Feel Proud?

The greatest thing I celebrate about learning to be present is that it's shown me the futility of living any other way than One Day at a Time.

Miranda, what have you done today to make you feel proud?

Thanks for asking. And I say to you this: Just done today. For tomorrow will take care of itself.

Habits

The next gem that came from living day by day as best I could, with a slower pace, was this: I became more awake to my daily habits. Which was both annoying and enlivening. Annoying because the 'ists' confirmed that every little choice we make has an impact. Who we are – and who we become – is made up of our everyday habits. So I had to face a few habits I didn't necessarily want to face, otherwise I was going to become an overthinking bag of crisps . . .

But if my daily habits were ultimately what made up my well-being (or lack of it), then changing some of mine for the better meant that I could take further responsibility for my situation. Sometimes this felt daunting, but in the main it was a glorious two fingers up to any helplessness that may have crept in over the years. It also meant I could continue to be kind to myself about the things that I couldn't change, things that were not my fault.

I got to a place where I could see some daily habits that were not serving who I was or wanted to be. This is where it was enlivening. I learnt from James Clear (whose book *Atomic Habits* is excellent for driving change) that habits are value-led. He talks about casting a vote for the person we want to be. Yay, there it was.

New habits were never going to be about doing things I felt I *had* to do – I once got sucked into experimenting with green tea first thing in the morning, and hated it from day one. I don't like green tea, and that's okay! I was also unnerved by claims that the only way to live fully and healthily was through an expert morning routine that included an hour of exercise, an hour of meditation and journalling, a nutty breakfast smoothie. No thank you says this HSP who needs a very gentle morning. Including hearty solid comforting food! But if I could form habits based on *my* values and *my* whys and *my* dreams, then new habits would be both exciting and possible. I honed my morning habits (this may sound simple, but any new habits take a couple of months to fully establish): brushing my hair, making my bed (confession – never did either daily before!), having a glass of warm water with lemon or ginger, going outside to look at the sky, smiling at something beautiful, saying a prayer, doing some shoulder rolls and pacing about a bit, then taking ten deep breaths before my large bowl of porridge and a big cup of tea, not looking at my phone until after breakfast. That's my morning routine. That's it. But it has a bit of everything I value – tidiness, movement, nature, faith, gentleness, tea! I will never get up at 5 am for a power hour (or three) of smoothies and weights and silent meditation. I know my body doesn't like exercising in the morning – it never did, even when I was a young athlete. And silent meditation is still not my way to be mindful. It's all about knowing how we uniquely tick, MDRC.

Tick, Tick, Boom

On which note, here's a little example from my life (well, it might as well be from my life considering this book is entirely about me . . .). It's about Guy Fawkes Night.

Every year in my twenties and early thirties when living in London, I would dread 5 November. Because I'm a little scared of fireworks. It's the banging – I don't like a bang! I really don't like it when you hear a firework launch into the night sky but don't know when it will explode so there's a moment of waiting to possibly jump with the fright of the bang. It's the same when I see a sign saying there is a gunshot in a theatre production. I can't concentrate – I spend the whole play wondering when the hell it's going to go off!

For about seven years I would trudge out with my friends to a fireworks display with thousands of people, pretending to enjoy myself, feeling foolish for hiding behind a friend and slightly screaming when they banged (the fireworks not my friend . . .). Not registering this trait about myself meant that I was always pushing my system to do other life things from socializing and beyond that it wasn't designed for, tiring it and stressing it (let's not forget, everything affects

325

our physiology). I feel sad that I wasn't awake to how I was feeling, instead overriding those feelings so spectacularly. Why wasn't I confident enough to share what I needed and wanted to do, how I wanted to socialize best? Well, you can't make your unique suggestions if you don't know how you uniquely tick.

Knowing how we tick is so important, MDRC. It's not picky, it's wise. The route to a reduced pot o' stress. Learning what time of day we best function at, how much sleep we need, what foods suit us, as well as the wider aspects of our personalities, such as introvertism or extrovertism, makes all the difference. They become like personal policies, helping with the big and little decision-making processes.

As I got more fluent in my personal 'tickery', a huge pressure lifted off me. I could just be, whole and complete, not rushing, not working out how to fit in. To me, that's wildness and authenticity and all that truly matters. Instead of trying to be that round peg in a square hole, I was slotting into my own hole very nicely (as it were).

If we learn how we tick, we tick along nicely and avoid ourselves going boom, like a firework – alight for a moment, making a splash, but fleeting. We all, I think, want to thrive at our best. And this, to me, continues to speak of kindness and gentleness to ourselves.

Examples Of Personal Policies For My Personal Tickery – Some Silly, All Sensible

- ◈ Phone completely off one day a week
- ◈ Walk every day
- ◈ Picnic once a month (picnics on sitting room floors allowed)
- ◈ Wear the same outfits chosen in advance when working on a big project (don't enjoy time spent on working out what to wear)
- ◈ Games night once a month (silly board-type games – nil screens)
- ◈ Go barefoot as much as possible
- ◈ Always say no to reading at carol concerts (I hate public speaking)
- ◈ Be naked regularly (not publicly – no public pubic-ness)
- ◈ Try or see something new or learn something once a month (have a mini adventure)
- ◈ Never host formal dinner parties and avoid dressing up for social occasions
- ◈ Try not to gossip or overshare
- ◈ Use email for admin and text for fun
- ◈ Do one thing at a time
- ◈ Save up for new Lego sets
- ◈ Have a feast day once a week (an apple crumble and custard for breakfast would be entirely permitted)
- ◈ Oh, and CELEBRATE regularly!

How often do you celebrate yourself, MDRC? I never used to. Now I celebrate myself all the time! I choose to tell someone if I feel I have done a good bit of work, asking for a 'go me'. I ask for applause if I do any washing-up because I hate it so! I think celebrating ourselves is a practical way to love ourselves. For me, though, it's also about humbling myself to the ordinary, maintaining gratitude at being able to do the simple things. I don't want to wait for the big events, like for a project to be finished, to celebrate. If life is made up of a sequence of the ordinary, then I want to celebrate them every day. If a family member unloads the dishwasher – whether they haven't for a while or always do it – surprise them, get a cake out, set off some party poppers! Celebrating another is a surefire way to make them feel loved . . .

What's Normal Anyway?

How you uniquely tick is never weird, MDRC, lest you ever considered it might be. If you're worried that your structures, your personal policies, your unique tickery is not normal, then, I say, what is normal anyway? Is there indeed such a thing? We have freedom to express ourselves how we are designed to, and perceiving there is a 'normal way' to be is a massive constraint.

If normal is having to be a member of a gym, then, as I always say, no thank you for THEY SMELL OF CROTCH. I shall exercise with a brisk walk in nature, plus my life doesn't require a six-pack to be fully operational.

If normal is always wearing make-up or the current fashion, then I say no thank you, I prefer au natural and am happy to wear socks and Crocs and a kaftan in public.

If normal is having to stick a job out until whatever is deemed 'the end' (e.g. a promotion even if I hate it), then I say no thank you for it's more important for me to follow my particular working path and choose trust over the treadmill.

If normal is having to have a birthday party every year, then I say no thank you for sometimes I just like to mark it with a day off on my own in my pyjamas.

If normal, when in a couple, from the age of thirty-five, is to throw a dinner party to feel part of 'society', then I say no thank you, I don't like to cook and prefer informal gatherings.

If normal is being in a couple by thirty-five, and it is considered strange to choose not to have children, then I say no thanks, you can fulfil mothering roles in many ways. And I would never settle just to be in a couple.

If normal is having to stay up to midnight every New Year's Eve and 'go large partying', then I say no thank you for I'm someone who needs a lot of sleep and doesn't want to start a new year, or any day, feeling rougher than I often feel. And for me, 'going large' is a sharing platter – for one.

If normal is having to have a specific career that will sound good when someone asks, '. . . and what do you do?', I say no thank you for I prefer to have experimented with lots of different things and call myself a 'dabbler'.

If normal is working until 8 or 9 pm every night as that's the way to be seen to be keen, then I say no thank you for my health and my relationships are more important.

If normal is not sharing emotions, then I say no thank you for I need and want to cry and laugh every day. I like to feel.

If normal is pretending you are okay when you are not okay, then I say no thank you. I will risk being vulnerable and sharing with a trusted someone that I am struggling.

If normal is being thin (still), then I say no thank you for my body shape isn't who I am and I want to love it however it happens to manifest due to various stages in my life. Plus, I like Nutella.

If normal is having the right stuff, then I say no thank you for I prefer my space to be really uncluttered and my T V and phone to function only as well as I need them to. I don't need anything new just because it's new.

If normal is sending abusive messages on Twitter to someone you don't know but dislike, then I say no thank you for I believe that everyone struggles and there's enough anger around.

If normal is for a woman to speak within a soft, restricted, elegant range, then I say no thank you for I want the confidence and freedom to speak deep, and to howl and wail when I need.

If normal is not being angry, then I say no thank you for sometimes I need to express irritability with my loved ones to then move on, and I want to be able to get passionate about what I believe in.

If normal is being able to survive on five hours' sleep a night, then I say no thank you for I can't and so there's no point me trying. I will have to turn down your job until I find one that meets my vital needs.

If normal is living in a city to be relevant, then I say no thank you for I often love to be in the middle of nowhere.

If normal is having millions of contacts in your phone, then I say no thank you for I would always prefer twelve very close friends and believe we only need one or two people we know we can ring up at 3 am in an emergency and we'll be okay.

If normal is having to excel in exams, then I say no thank you for I'm not academic and I excel in other ways. If I am not the best actor on a set (rarely, plus how can you judge art?), then I am certainly the most windy.

If normal is just being extroverted and loud, then I say no thank you for I love to listen and spend days in silence.

If normal is having to rush and be seen to be busy, then I say no thank you for I got the memo that there is an epidemic of burn-out and I don't want to work for someone who won't respect my pace when I'm naturally hardworking.

If normal is not being able to have a moment of silliness and cheekiness, then I say no thank you for silliness helps oil the joy in the world.

If normal is having to be normal, then I say no thank you for I don't think such a thing exists.

How you tick is perfect. Find your own rhythm. As Maya Angelou said, 'If you are always trying to be normal, you will never know how amazing you can be.' LOVE IT!

Keep It Simple

I might have considered anything resembling a simple life rather dull in the past. How naïve, patronizing and grand! Now it's all I crave, MDRC. All the learnings and practical steps of this treasure were taking me to simplicity.

I learnt that simplicity doesn't mean denial, it means intentionality. It means stepping off the merry-go-round to consider what I actually need and what particularly makes my heart come alive. My favourite definition of simplicity is this: 'Simplicity is letting go of things other people see as normal.' I find this so freeing (I knew it was okay not to have twenty-five scatter cushions on the bed!), and it made it even easier to stick to my personal tickery policies. An interesting thing I noticed about simplicity for me was its reduction of the inner critic – how with less stuff, fewer complications of busyness, there was less for that voice to criticize. As I got happier with what I had in my house, what clothes I wore on my back, what I ate, who I spent time with, how I worked, I was in line with my wild self.

We are not living a lesser life because we have a long list of unfulfilled desires. Simplicity means letting go of the ideal, because what *is* the ideal? When we're present and grateful and intentional and joyful, we have enough. We let go of the normal because what *is* normal? If we never get to Santorini, that's okay!

Dare Gently

I am more and more in love with the much-needed quality of gentleness.

The world still seems to value a 'never give up', 'fight, fight, fight', 'take things to the limit' attitude. But gentleness, too, is a way to never give up. A way to give yourself the calm, present, peaceful, humble attitude you need to change or be there for others. Isn't someone going to respond better to a gentle word rather than a telling off? How gently dare we go in a world that appears to have forgotten gentleness?

Going gently can be about many things, MDRC, but I found it most of a game-changer when applying it to how to go about a task. How easy is it to look at the mountain ahead and believe there's just no way, it's too much? Many of us are goal-orientated and want solutions asap, which of course fuels stress. It took me a while to see that the process *itself* is the goal, that I could enjoy the steps I was making here and now. Indeed, the practical way to describe gentleness is going step by step.

Dreams and visions are about the long road. If you ever find yourself putting the brakes on a process for fear or shame, MDRC, then maybe it will help to say to yourself, 'It's okay, sweetheart, what's the next loving right action?' It's a piercing weapon against the fear of the mountain to climb.

Gentleness leads to transformation because slowing down leads to transformation. And it all started with pottering for me!

'Enjoy the moment, because that is all you have. You are never going to arrive someplace else.' – Dr Wayne Dyer

I knew I had arrived in the now as I contentedly spent time with The Boy. Not because it was a heightened, exciting time getting to know him, but because I was now far happier in my own skin. I didn't need to run away, or make unnecessary jokes to avoid vulnerability, or flirt appallingly in an attempt to flirt the way I thought I 'should'. I was at home with myself, and I felt safe. I had been vulnerable, yet I felt dignified. I had shown him the silliest me, the irritable me, the farting me, the no-make-up me, the teary me, the deep me. I trusted fully that he was there because he liked me.

Was I feeling love? The moment I asked myself this, Patti got furiously jealous, leapt on to the sofa and sat right on my upper chest, bum almost in my face, declaring the area a kissing-free zone. Which was very poor timing!

Goodness, MDRC, had I found my person?

Go gently, Miranda. One day at a time.

Treasure Nine

Don't Fear the Setback

TREASURES PICKED UP: Perseverance, courage, tenacity, resilience, understanding, wisdom

PATTERNS SMASHED: Perfectionism, fear of failure, comparison, jealousy, helplessness, discouragement

WATCHWORD: Patience

SOUNDTRACK: 'The Long and Winding Road' by The Beatles

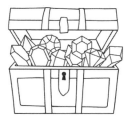

Don't Fear the Setback

Help, I'm Going Backwards

It wasn't until I suffered from chronic illness that I became familiar with the fear of the backwards step. I found I couldn't calmly and maturely surrender to any health setbacks. Instead, I was drawn to tantrum-ing like a toddler who'd just lost the ice cream from their cone (although, to be fair, it is a difficult setback for all humankind when the delicious, cool, creamy ice cream plops unrecoverably on to the beach or grass). Anything resembling a setback in my physical recovery and I would head towards the world of tantrum, airing petulant thoughts such as, *Why does this always happen to me?* or, *It's not fair*, or, *Everyone else has a much easier time of it* (that one is a terrible lie that gets a lot of us at some time or other).

I think partly why I wasn't adept at dealing with setbacks was because I wasn't familiar with failure. Let me quickly correct that, MDRC – not familiar with a *fear* of failure. I have had some epic fails. Certainly in my work life. I just didn't perceive them as such. In the main, I laughed them off. I will share a story based around an audition, which most of my acting friends shudder at, such would be their horror at the notion.

It was early on in my professional acting life, and I had a huge excitement in getting a part in a comedy drama starring Martin Clunes. My character was only in one episode, and appeared in two scenes, but this was big time for me. I did the scenes, felt I did them well, had a lovely and interesting experience. I was much buoyed by the acting affirmation and excited to have something new to add to my showreel. A couple of months later my agent rang to say that they were going to write up the part for the next series in which she would be a regular character. Right, now, this was *very* exciting. 'THIS IS IT!' I said to my agent. 'This could be a real break.' She was equally excited for me. She told me I was to have a meeting with the producers to discuss the part. *Of course*, I thought to myself, *they probably want some ideas from me, having played the character before.*

I went to the meeting and was told to wait in the hallway outside the office. The producer's assistant then gave me some pages of scripts. I thanked her and felt very smug, smiling proudly at the other people seated in the hallway. They all looked rather nervous, and I thought there must be an audition going on in another room as they were all studying and mumbling over their own scripts. I walked confidently into my meeting, did the reading, chatted about the part, and felt happy with how it went. The next day I rang my agent to ask what the next steps might be. She had to tell me the rather tricky news that actually I wasn't the only one auditioning for the part that day. There was a long silence from me. 'Hello? Are you still there?' my agent said. 'Yes, just trying to take something in – are you saying that I had to audition for a PART I HAVE ALREADY PLAYED?!' Now I thought about it, all the other people in the hallway were tall, dark-haired women of about my age. My agent explained that they would have been doing their due diligence because I didn't have that much experience and it was going to be a big part. Fair enough. She would call me in a couple of days and let me know the outcome.

To be honest, my agent and I were both sure the outcome would be that I would get the part. Considering it was a part THAT I HAD ALREADY PLAYED! But, if you haven't guessed already what might be coming – I DIDN'T GET THE PART!! Let that settle in, MDRC – I basically didn't nail the audition to play the part of myself!

I find it funny because a 'failed' audition doesn't unnerve me. It's not something that rocks my confidence or self-worth.

Setbacks are part of everyone's lives, but they only lead to stress and tantrums and deep disappointment if they relate to our most difficult experiences and fear-inducing limiting beliefs. I know people who are terrified of going bankrupt, so a month with a lesser wage packet causes genuine fear that they might spiral into financial difficulty. I have a friend who saw any relationship ending as an indication that she was best off alone, and she assumed people judged that she was impossible to be with and it was always her fault. I feared not getting better. When it came to any setbacks in my health recovery, I could not just pass them off as an interesting part of my life journey and sail calmly on, like I could following a disappointing audition experience.

I know that many people who have had similar illnesses – in particular energy-sapping ones like long Covid and ME – and those who have experienced the ghastliness of waiting for news of remission from any illness – will be aware of the fear of the setback. Often in energy-related conditions, these setbacks are known as a crash, dip or flare-up. Put simply, a time when the body feels like it has let you down, and you are 'back there' again. The fear of going backwards or symptoms coming back or having to go through something again, whatever it is, it is understandably tremendous.

Fear not, MDRC, there were pearls to be found as I dived into this treasure. I've got your back on the backwards steps . . .

Triumph And Disaster

'If you can meet with Triumph and Disaster
And treat those two impostors just the same . . .'
– Rudyard Kipling

I first became familiar with Rudyard Kipling's beloved poem 'If—' via my love of tennis. The above lines from it are inscribed at the entrance to Wimbledon's Centre Court. But it confused me. I never understood why it would be inspiring to players to suggest that you could treat Triumph and Disaster as the same. Surely Disaster is, well, a disaster. And why would he say triumph is an imposter?

Triumph is surely, you know, a triumph. It confused me for a long time.

I realized it was because, for some reason, I believed that life is meant to be lived with a solid upward trajectory, getting easier and simpler as we go on. That's winning, isn't it? It was hard-wired in me to say that disaster was an imposter and triumph was what I was striving for. It's probably back to the pattern of believing that life is about the avoidance of pain and a quest for happiness. But I know now that's the only surefire way to pain and unhappiness. We are not lesser, or unusual, for having an illness, or being at lower capacity than others around us for a time, or having limits, or struggling in our work or relationships. The expectation of a perfect upward trajectory of betterment and success can but lead to living under enormous pressure. That pressure fuels stress and means a setback can only be perceived as a disaster.

I lived so much of my life under the belief 'keep going because *then* I will be okay'. Hoping there is a time when it all comes together is, I'm afraid, MDRC, nonsense. There isn't a point we get to when we are suddenly ready, when we have the answers and can be perfect at everything, have it all worked out. But isn't that such a wonderful and enormous relief? Some people see their whole life as a mountain to climb, as if they can't rest until the very end. I strongly believe that's why we rush, push too much, because we are living under a limiting attitude or metaphor towards life. Mine used to be 'life is like wading through treacle'. Even saying that now and I feel a little stressed and tired.

I doubly trapped myself because I had not only lived under the belief of needing to get to a peak place to be able to 'start', but that my younger years were when all the success and excitement were meant to come. It's that nonsensical notion again that around thirty we need to 'have it all together'. If we think that, we will fear setbacks in our youth even more. The world shouts that it is in our younger decades when we should marry and have perfect, functioning relationships. When we need our working life sorted with a pleasing answer to '. . . and what do you do?' We are told that when we are young is when we look our best. Well, what about us handsome women who start to accept and grow into our looks in our forties, becoming fierce and fabulous and fantastic and foxy at fifty?! Why not start a marriage when you know who you are, and get a heavy injection of romance in mid-life? Sounds great to me. Wouldn't many dreams taste better if you reached them at seventy not twenty-five? I think so.

Life isn't an upward trajectory launched from an assured place in our youth. Life, by its very nature, is up and down. Life *is* bittersweet. Life *is* dark and light. (That's why joy is vital: it can be held within the darkness.) The highs and lows are all part of the mysterious path of life. Isn't the long and winding road a more interesting one anyway? I had no idea it would take me going to the Edinburgh Festival every year for eleven years, before I found regular enough work as an actor to give up temping. I would have a leaving do every July in my office job, convinced that in August at the festival I would get my break. Every September I would crawl back in asking for work. They eventually just kept the job open!

In the health setbacks I feared, I began to give myself a mantra, which helped many other aspects of my life: 'I will let my life unfold day by day, taking small steps towards my values, in self-compassion, with a bedrock of trust.'

That's probably the only way to find happiness. When we stop making a triumph mean we are a better person and a disaster mean that we are a mistake or a failure, we are immediately and lovingly letting ourselves up. And we become more compassionate to others' ups and downs.

Setbacks are a part of life – MDRC, remember that anyone we admire has likely had a story with many failures, mistakes, dangers, difficulties – and as I understood this, I wanted to find a way to accept the ones I feared. Do them well. In fact, if they are simply a part of everyone's life story, do I even need to call them setbacks?

When I was in the middle of a bad symptomatic setback, a fellow-sufferer-turned-recoveree-turned-therapist suggested I reframe it as being a lay-by. I was pulling in to listen to what to learn next, or have some rest, take stock. I wasn't going backwards. I found that comforting, and it sowed the important seed that setbacks always teach us something. They aren't pleasant. They feel icky and uncomfortable and frustrating and annoying and horrid. But the lay-by concept helped me to reframe them as an equally valid part of my life.

Hopefully I could try to see setbacks as part of the rich tapestry of my life and not the disasters I had previously labelled them, causing me stress as a result.

345

The Maturely Named 'Silly Setback Of Doom, Drudge and Despair'

Talking of tennis, athletes must be those most familiar with set-backs. I understand the mindset of a champion to be 'What do I learn from this?' and 'How do I go back into training to get stronger and reset?' They don't stop going to the gym and give up, believing they are now rubbish for having some losses. Losing is tough. The setbacks are tough. But if we view them the way a champion might, then they can be the greatest teacher in making us stronger, fitter and a better version of ourselves. They always breed resilience, courage and persever-ance. In fact, we need things to be challenging. Our mind and body need to be exercised to gain strength. Do you remember our lovely 'ist' John in the earlier danker part of the cave? The one boldly defining the concept of surrender for us? He told me that he had a client who was walking (literally and metaphori-cally) out of chronic pain, and she began to get annoyed when she started experiencing less pain on doing activities. 'Annoyed?' I said in astonishment. He said yes, explaining she no longer feared the pain flare-ups and ensuing fatigue crashes. She knew that experiencing them without fear was the only way she could rewire her brain off the stress response. And it was that which would heal her pain once and for all. She had started to enjoy the challenges, knowing that if you don't challenge yourself in little ways over time, and if you remain avoidant in the hard times, you can't become resilient enough to cope with the days that will be harder than you expected.

I found this very inspiring. But in the moment, completely and utterly infuriating! Because he told me this when I was in one of my more significant health setbacks. My angrily named 'Silly Setback of Doom, Drudge and Despair'. He was, of course, being helpful. But I was not yet fully surrendered to the inevitable ups and downs of recovery, instead putting my ideal timeline and trajectory on my story; anything that got in the way of that I still perceived as a 'disaster', with those low-energy, unhelpful thoughts including, this time, *I don't have it in me*. I spent a couple of weeks fed up and cross about having to be brave yet again.

However, I ended up proving the 'ists' – and ultimately myself – right. The setbacks/lay-bys of life are the times we learn what we need for the next part of our lives. Within my Silly Setback of Doom, Drudge and Despair, I learnt my heaviest of revvies in a long time (not science-based this time, you might be pleased to hear). Such a revelation that it unlocked a holistic understanding of all the treasures I had learnt. It was quite the defining moment for me ... Exciting times at the end of the cave, MDRC ...

Why We Need the Backwards Steps and My Exciting Next Heaviest of Heavy Revvies

In a brief moment of self-control within my Silly Setback of Doom, Drudge and Despair, I did some thought work on why – when I can be courageous, surrendered, calm, adventurous and joyful in other parts of my life – I was remaining so fearful of fatigue and sickness. I discovered a new root limiting belief. It was *the* root.

Firstly, I got to a thought I had met a few times before. I

was afraid of and frustrated by illness because it meant I was unable to do what I wanted to do with my life. If illness was a constant threat and frustration, then any little twinge of tiredness was inevitably going to freak me out.

I used the 'Five Whys' tool again. I wrote out the troubling thought, questioned it with a why, answered the why, and kept going until I, hopefully, found a root:

Fatigue stops me doing what I want to do.

Why does that matter?

Because, well, I want to be able to do what I want, with energy. I want to feel well.

We can't always feel well. Why do you always want to feel well?

Because then I will be okay.

Why won't you be okay if you aren't well?

A pause.

I hit upon something I had not yet uncovered. I got to the root below the fear of not being able to carry on and do what I wanted with my life.

The revelation was this, MDRC: being unwell and being unable to do what I wanted to do was scary for me. Scary because it meant that I might need to say no; I might need to cancel something, disappoint people and feel guilty for letting them down; I might have to feel sadness at missing out; I would have to face my vulnerability and weakness; I might have to ask for help; I might be alone; I might have to feel grief at not being able to find joy or gratitude.

It was only slowly dawning on me. 'Blow me down with a feather,' I said to myself (I like a 1970s camp saying). 'The treasures I have learnt in the dark cave of my suffering answer all those fears.'

Wow. I took a deep breath. It really was true. The treasures, and tools within them, *really do* answer those core fears. For example, if I keep connected and ask for help, accept my vulnerability and surrender, and on with all the amazing teachings in the treasures . . . then, I don't need to fear illness. Then . . . I have nothing to fear. Wow again. The treasures all help me meet my needs, and they really are the opposite of the world's shouts. Suffering can be a great teacher: how we grow and learn to be honest with ourselves and what's important to us, how to find the courage to go against the rules of the world.

Patti just bounded up on to my lap. A nice reminder of life unfolding. A year or so ago, if someone had asked if I was ready for a new dog, I would have crumpled into overwhelm. But here was this new fluff bundle of creation coming into my life at just the right time. Her full name being what became my watchword for this treasure – patience. Yes, I'm glad I developed a depth of courage and resilience in setbacks, but a much, much harder quality to develop, for me, was patience. I was not patient for patience. But I saw that impatience was not remotely kind or self-compassionate. Lying in bed with a fatigue crash and being impatient with my body was of course adding stress. Patience takes us to an even deeper love for ourselves, and others.

It would be easy to leave it there, but I want to make sure I take all the gems and treasures off the cave wall. So here are a few particulars I think we can learn from our friend the setback. First, though, I am going to have a calming song and sway break to 'The Long and Winding Road' by The Beatles . . .

Perfectionism

Gosh, I do love that song. I joyously swayed with imperfection and laughed at my failed harmony attempts!

Anyone with perfectionist tendencies will not enjoy the concept of a setback, let alone experiencing one. I can't speak with personal authority here, but I did read that for many it often comes from the past (little doesn't!), when, as children, they were led to believe that they had to perform perfectly to get approval and love in the family. They find mistakes very hard to cope with as a result. Plus, attempting perfectionism means you avoid being vulnerable or messy or weak (maybe that's where we all have it to some extent). If we are not comfortable in our own skin, we will do anything to avoid criticism or judgement. I think that's where procrastination often comes from too. It can feel safer to procrastinate than to start the project, put yourself out there and risk not being good enough.

It all goes back to the solution of truly belonging to ourselves and others to feel safe. As ever, if we try to disappear from ourselves to avoid judgement, the more we will disappear from our core values, distract from our why, and feel out of kilter and unhappy with who we are. If a setback in life brings a yucky feeling of discomfort, then we could perceive it as a glorious opportunity to dismantle whatever patterns we may have gone into to protect ourselves. And restart. The backwards steps are times to cultivate a gentle, loving patience with ourselves.

Do you insist anyone else around you is perfect in all they do? No, of course not. You just want those you love to have a go, try their best. We are all now, and always will be, a work in progress. We can never expect to be a perfect finished product. There lies misery if that's what we aim for. There is no shame in your cracks (if you pardon). In fact, MDRC, it's those cracks that make us love you, that help us connect with you, know you, understand you. Without them, you are a polite sheen. I continue to believe that we all want the real, true versions of each other to love and to hold on the long and winding road of our lives.

Stop Comparing

Now this was something I was marvellous at! Constantly comparing. If there is anything that will make a setback worse, or indeed cause one, it's comparison. Getting stuck in comparison can be caused by 'I should be further along' thinking, and then we wrongly judge where we are – or aren't – in our lives. It's all big fat lies!

It would be hard to talk about comparison without mentioning social media. It's too big an issue to go into here in full detail, but let's just say I wasn't very loving to myself in the Silly Setback of Doom, Drudge and Despair because I popped on to Instagram and scrolled. I thought I knew better and had rid myself of that habit. All my personal policies around it were out of the window in my doom! It led to a nasty bout of comparison. I happened upon photographs of friends in Capri, on a rooftop bar with a pool in London, by a river in Surrey, in a lovely pub garden, in their own garden with family eating ice lollies. Seeing all these I instantly felt more trapped by my limitations. I admit, I was jealous.

Luckily – before I could judge myself for feeling jealous – I had learnt that it is not only quite normal but points to why we might be restless and discontented. While uncomfortable to feel, it is a powerful emotional warning signal to remind us of our values. With freedom as one of my highest values, and adventure and nature as two of my great loves, all those images were hitting me where it hurt.

Comparison and jealousy also remind us that we are, in effect, judging others – assuming they are having the most marvellous time. Comparing our so-called small life with their apparent vast one. It's so easy to think the grass is greener. Which ends up not being a loving stance, as we don't see any fragility they may be holding or help they may need. I love this quote from Brené Brown: . . . if we're really paying attention, most people have a story that will bring us to our knees.' How quickly we forget that when we are stuck in comparison.

The best saying I know on comparison to help me stay kind is this: you cannot compare your insides with someone's out-sides. It's much kinder to ourselves and others to stay in our own lane, for there's only one of us, and the way we run our own race of life is unique to us. Don't get to the finish line scattered and exhausted. Fly through that line knowing you've raced in your lane and not against anyone else. If you try and get into anyone else's lane, it's only ever going to trip you up. Broken record alert MDRC – there's only one of you in the whole history of humankind. You need never compare yourself to another! Talking of records, I'm going in for another song break. Child of the eighties alert – I'm choosing 'We Belong' by Pat Benatar . . .

The Bamboo

I thought I'd rewired my brain enough for fewer tantrum-style fearful moments, but during my Silly Setback of Doom, Drudge and Despair – and the big dump of fatigue and ensuing neurological symptoms of old it caused – I was surprised how quickly old pathways reared. I went straight to, *Oh great, here we are back at the beginning. I expected myself to be so much better by now, this just shouldn't be happening.* The old wallowing hippo returneth! I went outside to lie on the grass. I set a timer for ten minutes in which I would slow my breathing and commit to surrendering.

There, I noticed a bamboo plant at the bottom of my garden. There was a dying brown branch and leaf entangled within a clump of fresh, green, healthy leaves. The dying branch was pulling them one way when they wanted to go another. It was a tug. I thought to myself, *What a horrible deathly grip that brown leaf has on those fresh green leaves that want to freely dance in the wind.* I was being shown a

353

beautiful and natural image of what the raging mind does. The raging, worried mind (the brown leaf) attacks healthy thoughts and values and pulls us away from the freedom and ability to be who we want to be in that moment. I walked over to pull the long, thin, dying branch away. It had wound around and choked the bamboo. I slowly unravelled it and pulled it up from its root. The healthy leaves separated from their entwining, seemingly exhaling, and moved to their natural position and settled. The wind died down and there was an extraordinary tangible peace. A tiny miracle in my tiny garden.

I already believed the treasures to be right and true, but to experience using them all in a ten-minute moment in my garden to placate myself was extraordinary. I detached from the thoughts that were constraining and oppressing me, I let the emotions move through, I was self-compassionate towards my experience knowing I could ask for help if I needed it. I looked around the garden at all that I was grateful for and found joyous. I was surrendered and in the moment, and I took the next gentle right action in line with my why. I now knew what I needed to do in any moment of chronic crisis. I knew what to do in the next ten minutes. All the treasures releasing me. Wow!

I chose to put the fear that I was going back to the beginning to one side, thanks to what I had learnt about thoughts. Mainly using the tool of listing evidence that spoke to the opposite of my fears, but each time I did, I came back to the present. Thank you Treasure Four.

Even in my worst health setback, I had to concede that this was crucial training. I remembered what I had learnt in the hardest part of the cave, in what I call the Sacred Second Treasure of Surrender: fighting and battling the brain and body would never work. If we can turn towards our difficult moments and emotions with kindness, knowing we are a wonky but wonderful work in progress, they can then dissipate. If things have permission to be, they tend to change, as 'ist' Steven Hayes says. Or they can exist without choking our well-being and joy. Simply be part of our story, not judged as worse or better than any other moment. Frankly, that feels like a well-earned superpower, particularly if it bred patience for this typically impatient woman who likes to tick things neatly off a to-do list and crack on!

Eventually I was able to say to myself, *Okay, I have got Lyme disease and it's been misdiagnosed for thirty-three years and wreaked havoc on my life. A lot of that has to be grieved and verbally off-loaded. But either I live with that and focus on it and feel sad all the time, or I accept it and see how I learnt from it and where it might take me next.*

I kept going back to my mantra: 'I will let my life unfold day by day taking small steps towards my values, in self-compassion, with a bedrock of trust.'

'Above all, be the heroine of your life.' – Nora Ephron

Push, Push, Push

Writing that title, I'm now thinking about someone giving birth. Apologies if you weren't and now you are. But – and go with this for I'm close to apologizing for potential naffness – I think we can birth a new version of ourselves with these treasures. As we love ourselves and become more honest with who are, the wild self that has become hidden in darkness is finding its place in the world. And much like childbirth, it is hard.

I'm now thinking of my time on *Call the Midwife*. Whenever we did a birth scene, I had more respect for those actors than on any set I'd been on before, or have been on since. The strain in acting giving birth was intense to say the least. After most of those scenes, when the director shouted cut, we would often end up with our head between our knees to try and stop the room spinning. The actress giving birth was spinning because she was literally hyperventilating to make the pain look realistic, and the midwives were either panting to encourage the right breathing or holding their breath nervously when handling an actual tiny newborn baby covered in baby oil. The fear of dropping that baby as you pretended to deliver it, knowing an anxious mother was around the corner looking at the screen, was full on. By the third or fourth take we were all jibbering wrecks! We had to find some laughs between takes to alleviate the pressure – thank you, Treasure Seven.

Although a birth of any kind will require some pushing through, and I learnt and relearnt the truth of the Sacred Second Treasure that any and every time I pushed myself *too* hard, an inevitable setback or fatigue dip ensued. I had to cultivate patience as I know change does not come from forcing and pushing. Not that I don't believe in challenging ourselves to lead to empowering experiences, but it has to

356

be the right empowering challenge. Never forcing. Forcing is scary; it's not kind. Thank you Treasure Two.

I always go back to what the next right loving step is. Take that. Because that's not scary. Then take another. Teeny-tiny steps so I don't freak myself out. (If I do ever freak out, I *always* go straight to joy or play – amazing, biologically proven armour for calm. Thank you again, Treasure Seven.).

We are allowed to pull out of the lay-by slowly, gently, like a kid at a party who takes a while to peek out behind their parent's legs before joining the others. Thank you, Treasure Eight.

If you try and push yourself into new habits too quickly, it will always backfire. New Year's Resolutions seem the obvious example. I know I told you I used to put dance classes at the top of mine every year in my twenties and thirties. Well, they were on top of a very long list. Dance classes are a good example of something fun and enjoyable and within my values, but my list included things that were frankly RIDICU-LOUS. I now resolutely refuse to get involved in New Year's Resolutions. I used to think a long list of changes to make would motivate, but I see now it's basically saying *how you are living is unacceptable, please change everything about yourself and become a completely different person on January 1st, if you could please, thank you.* So mean! The list included getting fitter, leaner and more toned; gaining numerous hobbies; being more socially 'acceptable' by hosting a monthly dinner party people would be talking about until the day they died. One year I included 'get regular pedicures'. I didn't have the money for regular pedicures, I have very ticklish feet so find them a bit of a weird social threat, and I prefer to be barefoot.

357

Why was I trying to become a regular-pedicure woman?! RIDICULOUS. With a long list of expectant change to become other than who you are in the moment, you are going to crumble within at least three days.

I knew I needed to change things slowly and incrementally because I matter and have a unique why, not because I felt guilty or lesser for not being a certain way.

Happy New Year.
Immediate expectations.
Happy One Day at a Time.
Happy Step by Step.
Deep exhalations.
A stroll.
A meal.
A smile.
A chat.
A stroke of a nestled dog.
Step by step.
Hands in earth,
in water,
on soft skin,
or keyboard.
That is all this step.
No pressures,
No judgements,
No goals.
Deep exhalations.
Each step slower, gentler, wiser.
The year so infused, now possible.

Never resolutions.
Only the next kindly promise,
simple to keep.
Deepening exhalations.

How Your Why Gets You Unstuck

I have just read of a seventy-four-year-old man from Bournemouth who is now in the *Guinness World Records* as the longest-serving lifeguard. He simply said that he loved the sea and loved helping people, so he had everything right there on the beach and hadn't felt the need to leave since he fell in love with it at sixteen. I smiled and exhaled with such joy on reading that. The simplicity of purpose with a why in all its glory.

It takes courage not to be discouraged. It takes effort to replace the exhaustion of a setback with meaning. But there's an ease with a why.

Keep Going, My Love, Keep Going!

After my big health setback, my body slowly returned to a more energetic and functioning place as I surrendered more and more. Little Patti and I were getting into a good rhythm – my morning routine now included 'playing parrot'. Before you jump to any unnerving conclusions, that simply means throwing Patti's toy parrot for her to fetch; it was a delightful injection of play to start the day. Things were feeling pretty good and then – and I almost dare not say this, MDRC, but I hope you have come to believe that we really *don't* need to fear the setback – there was another 'setback'! Life is indeed a roller coaster.

I was spending more time with The Boy from Bristol, and feelings were deepening. And then. We had to take a break. I know – ouch. There were a few reasons why we didn't know whether the timing was right to become an 'us'. It was hard. It hurt my heart. A lot I didn't know whether it was the end or whether circumstances might eventually mean we could continue getting to know each other. It was hard because that connection, safety, kindness, laughter, gentleness that had helped my recovery so much was suddenly not there. There was a brief ghastly emptiness from the disconnection. A remembering of past aloneness, and the longing I had dared to feel not to be on my own. With the tools to let those emotions be there and move through I didn't get stuck. Thank you Treasure Three. Ultimately, I trusted – similarly to whether I would get an audition or not – that it would work out for the best, and I had capacity to cope with either direction that it might take. The difference in living life when there is a bedrock of trust is immeasurable.

I was also grateful that I now knew, deep down in my soul, that even if I was going to be without those qualities via The Boy, they were the most important things in life to focus on. I was going to take responsibility for following those values I knew I needed, those which were curing my body of exhaustion and viruses. We can't farm out responsibility for ourselves any more than we can take responsibility for someone else.

I also got the chance to see that I had the patience for any setback that might come from a sore heart. Perseverance was hard won, but I had won it. And I had the other Patience – Patti the puppy.

Perhaps it would be Patti and Me, after Peggy and Me . . . My next dog husband . . . !

Keep Celebrating

The first thing I did with my sore Hart heart was to connect and ask a friend for a kind listening ear to share it all with. That was new. Thank you, Treasure One. That needed celebrating.

If we don't notice, acknowledge and celebrate progress and growth in our lives, we are much more likely to give up. Especially in the setbacks, I mean lay-bys. It's always best not to look back unless it's necessary to understand some patterns, or to acknowledge how far we have come. Looking back to celebrate yourself will propel you forward.

If we can accept life has downs, we are much more likely to celebrate the ups. When I expected life to be easy, it made it incredibly hard. After all these decades I finally understood that triumph and disaster could be treated equally. Thank you, Treasure Nine.

I believe we should start celebrating disasters as much as we do the triumphs. Have a setback party! Toast that we are now more courageous, resilient and persevering than ever.

Why do we only celebrate the good stuff with others? Life is easy when it's going well. It's in times of despair we need each other. And if we have setback parties, aren't we freeing others to feel okay about their crashes and dips?

I followed my own advice and had a sore Hart heart party with my friend. I reminded her that I was the appointed Royal Crumble Taster and she should go to the shops immediately and get me all the crumbles and all the possible toppings so I could go through them and decide the best combination. You know you have a good friend when they just curtsey with a 'Yes, my lady' and pop to the shops. She allowed my wallow with the first crumble as I missed The Boy so very much, but then she made me list my wins and all the progress I had made, using the remaining crumbles to celebrate and there-fore not to fully crumble!

Keep Kind

'Finish each day and be done with it. You have done what you could. Some blunders and absurdities no doubt crept in; forget them as soon as you can. Tomorrow is a new day.'

– Ralph Waldo Emerson

Everyone makes mistakes, goes back to old habits, gets over-tired, eats badly, self-sabotages, feels irritable and grumpy. As Emerson says, 'Finish each day and be done with it.' Is it kind, gentle or patient to ruminate over your mistakes and beat yourself up? The answer is no, MDRC, in case you were wondering . . . When we are making mistakes, we need more kindness.

Perhaps that is the greatest thing a setback/lay-by can help to nurture and nourish. Being as loyal and faithful a friend to ourselves as a dear dog would to us. On a day I am kind with myself, the day is approximately 8,867.56 per cent better (all statistics are made up). Thank you, Treasure Five.

Just Start, My Love, Just Start!

'"Are you ready?" Klaus asked finally.
"No," Sunny answered.
"Me neither," Violet said, "but if we wait until we're
ready we'll be waiting for the rest of our lives."'
– Lemony Snicket

Remember, MDRC, we are not waiting to feel more confident before we start. We are not striving to reach a place where we feel more settled and successful to start treating ourselves right or following our why. Make the best of where you are. Life is not about outcomes. Cease assessing and evaluating. Let it all unfold. Life isn't linear. However we feel, however it seems, we are always in progress.

Don't wait until you are ready.

Don't wait until you are fixed to start a relationship.

Don't wait until you are thinner or fatter to wear that dress.

Don't wait until you are better to find meaning.

Don't wait until you are confident to start working on a project.

Don't wait until you feel worthy to forge friendships.

Don't wait until you feel brave.

You will receive courage and worth if you start. Believe, then move out to receive.

And if like me you have moments of being paralysed by indecision, then may I offer this genius word of wisdom – decide! If it's a massive life decision that needs wise counsel from others, research and consideration, then obviously do that. But with the next steps, with the everyday things, just decide. And then stick with it. These decisions are not going to make or break you. A therapist once told me that doubt is a symptom of fear. Seeing that was hugely freeing for decision-making. If we put too much weight on decisions, thinking we are in control of how our life is going to go and that one decision might send us down a wrong path and affect our whole life, we'll be paralysed.

It's time to start now, where you are.

And it's never too late.

You don't need permission to move forward with your life.

You don't have to feel ready.

You are ready.

Just start, my love.

Treasure Ten

It's All About Love in the End

TREASURES PICKED UP: Humility, compassion, loving, generosity, connection, self-acceptance that you are loved even in your brokenness

PATTERNS SMASHED: Abandonment, selfishness, judgemental, disconnection, fear of rejection, ignoring compliments

WATCHWORD: Love

SOUNDTRACK: 'We Are the World' by Michael Jackson

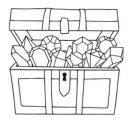

It's All About Love in the End

Hang On A Minute . . .

I was expecting my treasure gathering to end at Treasure Nine! I'd thought I was coming out of the cave blinking like an old but new fifty-year-old hefty foal ready to start life again. But before I could take my first step on to new ground, I was hit by yet another heavy revvy. I summoned my newfound patience and sat down metaphorically in the doorway to the cave (literally in my armchair overlooking my garden). I took a steadying breath, quietened my mind and listened to what this final revelation was trying to tell me.

It turned out to be quite the treasure, infinitely worthy of our time. And it's one that I will share as articulately as I can for our concluding chapter together (I'm missing you already, MDRC). Here goes . . .

I concluded that if, as I discovered while navigating setbacks in Treasure Nine, the solution to my core fears and problems was knowing that I could ask for help and meet my needs, *then*, I thought our most primal fear must ultimately go back to that of aloneness. Feeling alone means it's hard to get our basic needs met. We can't ask for help or cry with another vulnerably, be seen in our weakness, rest or find joy easily . . . and on and on the list of the previous treasure's healing components goes.

More than anything else, the treasures seemed to cure any disconnection and aloneness. To ourselves and each other. Which comes full circle back to our key identity—the need to belong. And, I suppose, MDRC, what that really means is LOVE.

I certainly had hints that, whatever else I was learning along the way, love was going to be the answer. If love – being loved and expressing love – is our ultimate identity, then isn't life learning to love? I feel I can truly say that my sense of what it meant to start again – after everything I had been through – is wholly about understanding myself, honouring that self, and showing myself love and respect. In turn, I find I have the capacity and desire to love outwards, in a wholly intentional way.

Humans are neurobiologically wired to be loved and to love. Everything else is noise.

When we take away the noise. When we take away the worldly non-serving desires. When we take away all the stuff we crave. When we take away the success we desperately strive for. When we take away all the takeaways we want to eat (I just wanted to say 'take away takeaway'). When we take it all away – and it is indeed all taken away from us in the end – at that point, at the end of our time, I feel sure we will know that all that truly matters is if we loved and were loved. There's a reason the top regret of the dying is what it is. There's a reason we so readily want to say 'just be yourself' to our loved ones – we see who they are, their capabilities and wondrousness, often before they do. Setting yourself and others free with love, is for me, a life of meaning. Our best legacy. We fulfill our human design.

We may have loved through the advice we gave, a smile to a stranger, money we donated, employment we offered, working hard for something or someone we believed in, parenting, looking after or rescuing an animal, encouraging someone, listening, reminding someone to look after themselves and the planet, creating a piece of work or a garden. There are myriad ways we can show love. I think of the friends who organized a fortieth birthday for me (*Strictly* themed, obviously) because they insisted I was celebrated. Or the colleague who knocked on my door unannounced when I was recovering from a back injury and simply stated 'Stay put, I'm coming to clean your kitchen!' Or my brother-in-law who read to me when Lyme symptoms meant concentrating was too hard.

It's so difficult to describe the feeling of love. And who on earth am I to try, if some of our greatest poets have not always been able to! Instead, I will offer up a practical suggestion for those who may have had to learn or relearn the concept when traumatic experiences may have taken away the belief in it. For me it started in my head – to trust that I was loved and loveable just by existing. Helped by my faith. Then, to move that knowledge to my heart, it was about making the effort to look for this indescribable, elusive force and power at work amongst us. I realized that for so many years I had never really let the kindnesses of friends and family truly sink in as proof I was looked after. I had been too focused on the invisible physical symptoms I was dealing with. So, I started small. If I noticed a beautiful flower, I would thank such an extraordinary ordinary thing that I would previously have dashed past, as loving provision – some beauty just for me in my day. I would notice a hospital receptionist's kindly eyes and smile as she told me that everything was going to be all right, and consciously let myself feel loved by it. Even if the sun shone on a day that felt important to me, or I had a cosy sit down with a delicious hot chocolate on a winter day, I would reframe it all as love. Let alone when someone helped me out or gave me a gift, or a compliment. In noticing all the forms of love around in each day I began to rewire away from any negative thoughts that might have crept in to say I was alone in my problems, or that life was just too tough. I believe there is so much love for us in this world to draw upon, and when we notice its effects in our lives, we naturally want to give it to others where we can.

If my attempt to reflect love in a practical way doesn't res-onate, let me sow a little science of love. I think we've got it in us to do a final bit of the academic pondering MDRC . . .

Get this: Dr Leaf tells us that recent neuroscientific research demonstrates that when we are operating as who we truly are, the brain releases chemicals including oxytocin, which, as she says, literally melts away negative, toxic thought clusters (e.g. the inner critic) so that the rewiring of new nontoxic cir-cuits can happen (e.g. the feeling of self-respect and worth). This chemical also flows when we trust, bond and reach out to others. So, choosing to operate through love can literally wipe out fear. I mean, wowzers.

It starts to get way above my pay grade to delve much deeper, but I just about understood this next cool bit because of what I had learnt in previous treasures: human biological evolution shows us that our foetal brain leaves us entirely dependent upon others. It's vital that we have nurturing, loving influences surrounding us because our brain doubles in size during our first year. It's why the first few years of life guide how we will fare psychologically and socially. But the 'ists' confirm that we can change and overcome any negative effects from childhood via our friend neuroplasticity. Things really can change for us all, MDRC, whatever our start in life.

Science shows us that our health improves as we love ourselves and each other. Feeling loved means we feel safe, and feeling safe keeps our nervous system functioning in homeostasis. Which, as we now know is essential, as it's our nervous system that interacts with our other key systems (immune, cardiovascular, endocrine, muscular, lymphatic and respiratory) so that our organs may function effectively.

There you have it. Love isn't just a nice idea. It keeps the mind, brain and body well. Again, wowzers.

I've heard many people say, 'I just want my kids to be happy.' And that's often our instinct – as long as our loved ones are happy . . . (Of course we want that.) But what if they can't be happy for some reason? What happens if they lose their health? What happens if their marriage comes unstuck or they lose a partner? What happens if their dream job never pans out? What happens if they live in a country in which a war breaks out? We might not understand the hardship and cruelty that continues in this world, but we know it's there. I wonder whether wanting ourselves and our loved ones to be happy is a stressful business? Happiness can be taken away at any time. When we say we want our loved ones to be happy, perhaps what we are really saying is that we want them to know they are loved, and we hope there is also icing on the cake in terms of good jobs and fun holidays and wonderful relationships and all the excitement, wonder and beauty this world has the capacity to give. But that's just the icing. If that's taken away, we need a cake. If you really want some-one to be happy, then you want them, ideally, never to feel insecure and unconfident in who they are; you want them to know they are good and loved. And then you will know they are going to stay healthier, and to live their life as well as they can, loving others, despite what circumstances they may find themselves in.

That's it.

Does anything else *really* matter?

(And let's just make it very clear that romantic love, let alone an idealized Hollywood version of it, is an *infinites-imal* part of the force of love. That kind of heady romantic love isn't lasting – anyone in a marriage will tell us that! It's the best friendships in all their guises that ultimately pro-vide the safe, nurturing, authentic love. And in a moment of crisis that might just be the holding of a hand with a stranger (turbulence on an aeroplane, anyone?). By the way, I prom-ise I will get around to telling you what happened with The Boy from Bristol before the end of book.)

Sitting in the doorway at the end of this almost decade-long cave, I can look back at the treasures again. Suddenly, it's clear that each one is a guide to loving ourselves and others better. Not a single one fails to fit within that remit. Each

374

treasure is kindly. Upbuilding. Encouraging. Each one adds another layer of how to feel and give love. Each one smashes a pattern of unimportant noise. Coincidence? When it's been proved we're wired to love and be loved? Not to me!

I once heard my young niece say, when listening to her grandparents explain the history of warring countries, 'Why doesn't everyone just get along? I don't understand it.' Well, quite, and indeed! Whenever I've had discussions about faith, it's always ended up with the simple agreement – mystery of faith aside – that if everyone did unto others what they would have done unto them, the world would be a better place. And again, quite, and indeed!

As we love ourselves more, we love others more, as we love others more, we love ourselves more, and a lovely loving loop creates more and more individual and universal wellness.

Well, that was all worth sitting down for. Thank you, cave. You came from suffering, and you were miserable to step into to start with, but you really did teach me all I needed to be well and start again. I am now less averse to the saying, 'The only way out is through'!

I wish I could end it there. But then . . . Love isn't simple.

We live in a world – and I find it agonizing to confront – in which love can be twisted, manipulated and confused, thereby stripping people of their trust in the very thing they need most. And so, MDRC, I want to share with you some final patterns which, when smashed, can help to bring us back to a place of love.

Blocks To Love

It might be a little sad – but perhaps also a relief – to know that it's not a quick and easy flick of a switch to 'be yourself' and 'love yourself to love others'. It will always be something we have to learn, relearn, discover and uncover.

My clear block to love was the old over-independence thing. The classic 'I will go it alone and not ask for help' pattern (you know me, MDRC!). Of course that trait took me further away from love. Of course it wasn't fair on myself or others wanting to love me.

Isolating is another block to love. There it was again, making ever more sense to me. And I hope it makes sense to you too now, MDRC: if as humans we are wired to belong, then not belonging and being rejected is our greatest fear. Isolating can then feel a safer option than risking asking for help and being rejected.

Fear of rejection is ultimately where all the blocks to love stem from. A fear of rejection is no doubt behind independence and isolating as well as other blocks we might recognize from day-to-day living: FOMO (fear of missing out) or cliquiness – (another way to try to belong is to cling to a gang as fiercely as possible.)

Other blocks: feelings of insignificance and unworthiness, distrust of others, pride, control, comparison and competitiveness (if we feel better than another, especially if we can measure that somehow, we are potentially filling an unconscious gap of love).

And we can't forget our old friend people-pleasing. Seeing it within the context of this treasure, it was clear to me how people-pleasing is driven by fear and not by love. Fear focuses on our problems. We aren't able to 'go out and be a blessing', as a dear friend of mine's mother used to say to her when she was a child, if we are riddled with insecurity, desperately searching for approval.

My favourite definition of humility, which comes from author and vicar Rick Warren, is that it's not thinking less of yourself, but thinking of yourself less. I saw that if I thought well of myself, believing I was inherently loved and approved of even when I naturally made mistakes, I was freed from many habits and fears. Which meant I could think outwards and love better. This also helped me to feel more forgiving towards others. If all the awkward and disturbing and inelegant ways we can communicate with our fellow humans are ultimately so as not to be rejected, then we are all just trying to cope with the same condition.

I found an interesting and unexpected block to doing an act of love recently in a moment of shyness, which perhaps in itself comes from a fearful, self-focused place. I walked past a woman on the street who was hauling a very heavy outdoor table on her own into the café in which she worked. I heard that wise, still, small voice within whisper to me, *Ask her if she wants some help.* What did I do? Smiled and walked straight past. (Occasionally I feel shy about the weirdest

377

things.) I forgave myself for it because despite all we might know, we're always going to be those wonderful, weird, wonky works in progress! But I do wish I had boldly done this tiny act of love that day – we might have got into a fun conversation or she might just have needed a small act of kindness to renew her faith that there is good in this difficult world of ours. She may of course have told me to **** off, but I would still rather have offered! Doing the loving thing is, in my experience, always the right thing.

On the more ridiculous end of the spectrum, I can see that some of my cringeworthy experiences might have their root in an attempt at ingratiating myself. To give ourselves a silly breather, I think of the time I met Jack Dee as part of an audition. We were all partaking in the slightly awkward informal chit-chat before reading from the scripts, and got on to where we lived. When Jack said he lived in Wandsworth, I found myself saying, a little too loudly, when the conversation wasn't really in my general direction, 'Weird, so do I!' I didn't live in Wandsworth, MDRC! I have never lived in Wandsworth. What happened?! An impulse to join in, to be friends with Jack? Obviously, it backfired for he then said, 'Whereabouts?' and I replied, 'Fulham.' To which he had to say, 'That's not Wandsworth.' I nodded in the awkward silence, wanting to do anything to have the powers of invisibility.

And now I'm thinking of the time that I went to a school disco with bread rolls under my bra straps to look like I, too, was part of the eighties fashion brigade who all had cool shoulder-padded tops on. Awkward when one bun fell off on to the dance floor . . .

I think of the time . . . In fact, I won't go on. It's another book. One I have already written. If you want more awkward shenanigans of a young woman, then read *Is It Just Me?* by – ME! It's all in there. All the wonderful and woeful ways we may try and fit in.

It's Everyone Else's Fault!

A rather yucky trait I had to understand in myself was having times of being a harsh critic. And I don't mean to myself this time. Let's just say, I had to delve into how I occasionally feel quite strongly towards other people in not the kindest of ways! Still, now, there are times when I am on the road and EVERY-ONE is a far worse driver than I am and doing EVERYTHING WRONG and definitely NOT QUICK ENOUGH! I will be shouting at them and telling them so (from the safe confines of my soundproof vehicle to avoid any confrontation . . .). I'll also admit I've had a full-on argument with a satnav before, calling her a 'screechy idiot', raising my voice as if she were a real person, saying things like, 'No, I can't turn left, actually, you've got that wrong,' and, 'No, I am not at my destination yet. Stop telling me I am, you stupid arsehole.' Or, there are times when the dear people behind the café counter ARE NOT GETTING MY TEA QUICK ENOUGH. Or heaven forfend someone gets their order before me – they become a wrong 'un by asso-ciation! I was pleased to discover that, in most of us humans, as much as an inner critic can develop, so too can an outer one . . . Most definitely another block to love. And it can become a little more serious than the general middle-aged grumpiness I allude to above (though even that never feels good at the end of a day). At least I now know when I am arguing with a computer-ized voice that I need to consider I am not giving myself enough space or rest, at the very least.

I learnt from our lovely 'ist' Gabor Maté that the outer critic might manifest in attitudes like judgement, accusing, wanting perfection in others, being passive-aggressive, road rage (oh dear . . .), anger at people who don't conform to your way. I came to understand they are often signs of unconscious inse-curity and unmet needs. It can be easier to get caught up in the drama of somebody else's issue than to face why we might be reacting that way and turn inwards. By criticizing outwardly, we justify to ourselves that other people are bad eggs. It's a clever ploy against shame, for starters. Being angry and judgemental towards others can make us feel that much stronger.

It's slightly annoying to have learnt that when you become irritable and judgemental of others, you are most likely being triggered by your own vulnerability. Byron Katie would be my go-to 'ist' to look up if you struggle with angry responses to others. Though be warned, she will tell you that if you are irri-tated with another, there's a 99.9 per cent likelihood it will be because they have mirrored some behaviour you don't like in yourself. When you are cross with your partner, it would be a lot easier and happier an outcome if it was all their problem and nothing to do with us. Just simply that they were being a total twerp and we remained innocent and perfect! (good word – twerp.)

Kill With Kindness Because People Don't Enjoy Being A Twerp!

My general feeling is that most people don't enjoy being a twerp! I don't think most people's intention on waking up is, *Hurrah, another day to be as much of a nightmare as I possibly can to as many people as I can and cause as much disruption and unpleasantness as I can – that's going to make me feel GREAT.* I'm sure there are some people who have simply become twerps, and their twerpery has become their identity, and they have decided to stay twerping about. You can't win them all.

I remember once advising someone who had a colleague who was making their time at work very difficult and demanding, 'Have you tried to kill with lightness and kindness?' It's scary to be confronted with twerpery, and we can forget that the person doing the twerping is still a human, and likely a fragile one. To deal with their fragility they may act tough, defensive or argumentative. The concept of admitting insecurity is still abhorrent to many. They can often do anything to keep any defectiveness hidden (back to the fear of rejection), even if they end up being labelled a twerp of the highest order.

If we forget that we can placate someone who is acting up with kindness, then we can so easily end up gossiping about them (I long for less gossip among adults), and turning them into more of a monster. If we remember that it could be their inner critic gone mad, we can see a real human under the twerp-ness.

Disarming bad behaviour with kindness can often stop it dead. It's hard for someone to fight back when they are being treated gently and with compassion (probably because that's exactly what they need). Their defences can come down as they are praised, encouraged, listened to, asked how they might feel more comfortable. Which is exactly what happened with my friend's colleague. And we certainly have to be kind to ourselves, even if we've been a twerp. Because we can try our best but still end up in an argument with an automated satnav . . .

I'm happy to share a meltdown moment in lockdown when, in the absurd stage of wiping down all deliveries (such was my fear of the virus), a lovely and exhausted delivery man sneezed as he approached my open front door. I reacted by slamming it in his face, nearly taking his nose off, and shouting, 'Get further away, NOW. That really is quite selfish of you to keep working if you are getting sick.' He shouted back that he was working his socks off getting food to people and was suffering solely from terrible hayfever. I immediately felt bad. In that moment I was just scared, and I behaved in a bad and judgy way as a result. What a twerp. (We did make up.)

Moments of twerpery can of course be funny too. I had such a moment of late. I was taking little Patti around the block for an evening walk and I was listening to some music on speaker on my phone. I rarely do that, but I don't like wearing headphones, and there was a song I needed to listen to for work and no one was around so I thought all was okay. It made for a jolly walk as I sang along to the tune and a jaunty little swagger developed (such a natural mover, MDRC . . .). The song, I should add so you can get the full and mildly eccentric picture, was 'Under the Sea' from *The Little Mermaid*. Yup, classic. As I was sauntering along, a man got out of his car and started whistling. I thought he had heard my music and was joining in. *What a lovely little interconnecting life moment*, I thought to myself, and in full twerping glory I turned up the volume, made eye contact with him and danced a bit more towards him . . . until I realized he was standing still, frowning and staring at me, clearly wondering what the hell I was doing invading his personal space. That's when I realized he had his headphones in and was not whistling to *The Little Mermaid*, but to whatever he was listening to (probably not a Disney score). I would like to try and say this was me making a point that headphones are isolating, and if only we could engage with each other more than with our phones . . . but although there is a point in that, in this case, I was simply being a full-on TWERP!

I didn't mind. I laughed. The more we know and love ourselves, the more any kinds of idiotic moments become a joyous, celebratory part of our life rather than embarrassing or shameful. (Kill ourselves with kindness.)

P.S. I have chosen to believe he backed away because he feared he might fall head over heels in love with me and my swagger . . .

One

This section is called 'One' because I couldn't name it 'Oneness'. The word oneness makes me cringe. It gives me the heebies as much as the thought of putting cotton wool in my mouth (who discovered how bad that was?!). Yet, it's where I'm heading. To the fact that we are all one. Urgh – why does it make it sound so naff? I feel the same about the phrase 'common consciousness' as part of explaining we are all united. They are both only saying that we are in this life together, so I should love the words. (Like I have begun to love the word 'moist'.)

> 'If we have no peace, it is because we have forgotten that we belong to each other.' – Mother Theresa

Being neurobiologically wired for love and belonging means we are all connected. That's why it's so painful to deal with conflict of any kind. It keeps going back to this glorious final revelation of a treasure – that the root of our human condition is the fear of rejection due to our need to feel love for survival and health.

It also concluded with clarity that all the masks we wear – whether masks of fear, fighting, fixing, judging, self-criticism, busyness, people-pleasing – have been worn to hide ourselves and the feelings and experiences we don't feel we should be having, all in order to fit in and belong.

Steven Hayes, in his other brilliant book *A Liberated Mind*, wrote, 'Genuine self-esteem is soft and open to our own flaws; the kind built on pretence is rigid, defended, and rejecting of self-honesty.' Wow, 'rejecting of self-honesty' really hit home. Our masks are all about increasing our self-esteem with images and stories and goals (often so far away from who we actually are) to feel better about ourselves.

All we really want from each other is to be ourselves, and to get to know the real people around us. All our different skills and different ways and thoughts and visions and missions and dress sense and body shapes and humour and perspectives and stories. All different, but united in our shared humanness. Not a homogenous mass of polite masks. *'Love takes off the masks that we fear we can't live without and know we cannot live within.' – James Baldwin*

Because we are one.

When we realize our existence works because of love, we can look outwards, beyond the self, knowing we are part of something bigger. When we want to be part of something bigger than ourselves, old 'noisy' desires can seem unsatisfying, and a freedom from approval, comparison and the need to succeed can follow.

We are a small but significant dot in a big ocean of love. To make an ocean we need every little drop of water.

Because we are one.

You are a lovely drop of water!

Love-Hacks

Here are a few love-hack suggestions as we come to the end of our time together:

- ◈ Treat everyone as if they like you and notice how different that makes you feel.
- ◈ Repeat regularly to yourself that you are loved. Love casts out fear. As you start to love yourself, fear of how you are being perceived can start to vanish.
- ◈ Know that if you can love others, you have the capacity to love yourself. Why do you love them? Because you just do. They bring you joy. Because they exist. You are no different.
- ◈ John O'Donohue said we 'mistake glamour for beauty'. You do not get your worth from how you look. Who you are is what people love.
- ◈ Name three things at the end of each day that show that you were good enough. Think of what you would say to a friend to avoid judging yourself.
- ◈ Compliment more. I experienced such a generous compliment once from the one and only Mary Berry. Someone so loving she's basically a cosy cup of tea and a cushion in human form. (And I love her for also embracing the word moist.) She held my hand, looked me directly in the eye and said, 'Miranda, you are beautiful. Don't ever put yourself down thinking you are anything else.' (I think she was worried I believed some things that had been said in the press about my looks.) I skipped energetically through the rest of the evening I was so high on the compliment. An authentic compliment can be life-altering at the right time. I truly believe that.
- ◈ The more good we see in others, the more good we see in the world and ourselves. It's always good to practice looking for the good.

- ◈ Keep getting to know yourself and how you uniquely tick and what you uniquely love to do.
- ◈ Check impulses, desires and motives to see which are more loving and compassionate for yourself and others.
- ◈ Repeat and repeat and repeat the truth that there is only one of you in the whole history of humankind therefore you are uniquely valuable.
- ◈ Do something to make yourself feel proud, like an act of service to another.
- ◈ Encourage each other to be the best version of ourselves – but without pressure and exacting standards. Repeat after me, MDRC – we're always a work in progress! I often ask a couple of inner circle non-judgemental friends, if they see me not being a good version of myself, to tell me and help me get back on track. As Brené Brown put it, 'When we stop caring about what people think, we lose our capacity for connection.' It's not that we should be swayed by fear of what others may think, but it's not actually loving to dismiss good feedback. It's a safer stance to go, 'I don't care what you think, I just do me, deal with it.' But if we are confident with ourselves, we don't need that position, and we can listen objectively to feedback, and be flexible for what others need.
- ◈ Know you can love with your brokenness. We feel whole if we accept we are loved even if we are a mess, instead of wearing masks to try not to be a mess. We are all interconnected in our mess and our stress. What alleviates both is being available to help each other with both. It is in our honest brokenness that others want to love and understand us – then we have the skill to do that for others.

If I'm Being Honest . . .

I haven't spoken much of my nineteen-year-old self recently, which is intriguing when that sense of freedom she had was so often a constant nagging, grieving nostalgia to (now) middle-aged me. I believe it's because I have reclaimed parts of her that were missing, particularly since joyously getting my joy back. Through the treasures, my honesty and authenticity were able to grow. I became closer to her and therefore my wild self.

It's not like I have spent my life deliberately lying, but what the treasures of my darkness showed me is that all the micro-lies are why I became, in many ways, untrue. All the following-along with the crowd when my heart was screaming for the opposite direction, all the agreeing with conventions that deep down didn't suit, all the accepting of values that didn't sit right, all the nos that needed to be yeses, all the yeses that needed to be nos. They all added up to not being fully honest with myself.

You cannot be authentic if you don't know who you are – it's honesty that gets you there.

It's only now that I understand how I honestly function.

I think that this is why I walked through the cave. The woman I was to greet on the other side was the loved and loving version of myself. I was going to be vulnerable and get it wrong and be judged and misunderstood, but it wouldn't matter. I was now solid in who I was and the meaning of my life, leading to a freedom and joy for me with my knocked knees and thinning hair as I obsessed over my eclectic selection of dogs and farmyard animals and Lego sets!

I needed to go into the cave and focus on myself for a bit, so that I could become free to focus outwards. I was starting the journey to put others before myself. With that came the most robust sense of freedom and joy yet.

And now, I can walk away from the cave.

I am home now.

I belong.

And it feels wild and free.

Shall We Dance?

Why are you hiding, my soul?
My little one,
I see you at the bottom of my heart
In the dark,
Daring to peek out.
The light seems daunting now
But I will hold you.
Why have you been hiding, my soul?
Below all the layers I have been trying to solve,
You were there.
I see you now.
I pick you up.
It's time for you to take over,
To soar,
To reveal yourself.
I am ready to dare.
Can we dare
To pick up the pieces,
Throw away the masks
And dance?

– Me

PART THREE

Wild and
Home

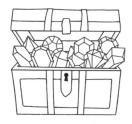

The Final Goodbye

The many moments, metaphors, experiences and stories of the last decade have culminated in one key understanding – I have finally come home to my wild self. It is a sure feeling, but I am less sure how to *express* it. Part of me wants to shy away from even attempting to. If my final musings feel scatty, or inadvertently poetic(!), then I hope at least some truths within them land or make sense. For we have come this far together, My Dearest Reader Chum, and I would be remiss not to complete the story with you. For this is, after all, our goodbye. Plus, there's one part I'm dying to tell you.

I used to hate goodbyes, but now I see them as a chance to thank the person, moment or experience; I'm more grateful if something is harder to bid farewell to, for it means it was ever more precious. Mostly, the sting of my goodbyes has lessened because I'm able to look ahead with trust not trepidation. With an inner quietness that provides me strength. That is certainly a new beginning, and I'm assuredly not sad to say goodbye to any of the past striving and stress. Oh gosh, have I gone 'poetic' already?!

I have, in the main, said goodbye to ME caused by Lyme disease. I will always to some degree carry my past – but it no longer defines me. When it does sometimes direct me, such as having to manage fatigue, then I rarely fear it (it's just blooming boring and tests my patience!). Mainly because I now understand the mind–body connection and have hope for a full recovery. With the discipline to keep working on the tools that reduce the stress response, and the surrender to release control over what I can't, my ordeal is over.

(This doesn't mean life becomes plain sailing. It doesn't mean that life no longer involves duty and sacrifice and hard work and perhaps some more dark caves ahead. But it does mean that my ability to deal with the trickier parts is greatly increased, and there's a chance my degree of suffering will never be as high as before. Even if I get sick again.)

As I continue to slow my pace, rest, notice what habits I need to remove and intentions I need to cultivate, as I detach from judgement and criticism, manage my energy, celebrate regularly, stay grateful and playful, follow a pressure-less purpose to love (accepting I will fail in some way everyday), I am letting go of the patterns that never served me. The old ways that cause harmful stress are dying and shriveling up (literally neuroscientifically – yay!).

I like to say this: if we smash patterns, we become pattern-smashers for ourselves and others, and then we become a smashing pattern of who we are meant to be, and not a replica pattern smashed by the world. (Really quite pleased with myself with that.)

Each day, I may have to say another goodbye, to an old pattern not yet undone or an old reaction not yet completely rewired, but I know, too, that there is the possibility of renewal.

I have new norms to say hello to.

Anchored

One day, not too long ago, I watched the 2022 film *Pinocchio* by Guillermo del Toro. One scene in particular surprised me, for it gave me a realization of quite how much I needed not only a structure in my life, but clear guidance to follow. It was an epiphany that without that structure and guidance, I would once again be trapped and buffeted about by others' opinions, losing the true wild self that I had discovered in my cave time.

MDRC, that's basically what I want to say here, at the end of our time together:

Being home is being grounded in the truth that we are wholly loved, which sets us free to live honestly, not shaped by the world's ways or the hurts of our past experiences. That, to me, is being our wild selves. And, as we now know, the more authentic and wild we are, the more lovingly we naturally respond to the needs of ourselves and others.

Boom, nailed it. *Drops mic and gallops into the sunset . . .*

I'm back. I want our final goodbye to be longer, MDRC!

Back to the film . . . When Pinocchio first emerged it was via a fabulous song in which he expressed his complete delight and joy at meeting everything in the world for the first time, from a broom to a clock to a wooden wheely stool. It was wonderful – and sparked this worn-down adult to, as ever, yearn for the excitement and wonder of childhood discovery.

But within this lovely scene, Pinocchio was also demonstrating utter chaos. He did what he wanted with a glass bottle he came across – namely, smashing it. He used a hammer with disastrous consequences and fashioned a rug into a cape. He was playing, he was joyful, he was freely doing whatever he wanted, but he wasn't considering the ruinous effects. When I tapped into this chaos of someone not understanding how to act with another, not understanding how to be kind, how to love, basically how to be human, it felt a clear picture of what life can feel like without a container of simple, loving rules to follow. An ineffective puppet with no strings. A bumbling, middle-aged woman without her treasures.

I used to think that to have strings – aka 'rules' – would mean confinement. Now I believe that I don't work at my best if my mission is simply to do whatever I desire. Being boundary-less in that way creates more stress than feeling anchored to a way that gives me meaning.

I no longer subscribe to patterns that cage me but instead I look to the treasures that free me. These ten treasures, I have learnt, are my anchor. My puppet strings.

The strings are long – I am not remotely confined or limited – but I am tethered to values that serve my best wishes as well as those around me. Although I will no doubt make some wrong choices, and some decisions might still hold worry, I have less fear that I will go so far off course as to smash up the place Pinocchio-style in immature confusion.

I need my strings, my anchor, my treasures (choose your analogy, MDRC) to avoid chaos.

The treasures keep me on a path within which there is more freedom than I ever experienced without them. If I'm feeling anxious, unsettled, confused, insecure, egotistical, then I know one or more of my strings has been cut loose, and I need to work out which one and tie it back. I need to find more patience or gentleness or joy or acceptance or self-compassion. And I need to do so before I reach for crisps and a box set!

If I lose a touchstone and veer off my path, I now know how to calm the chaos. This meant a clear goodbye to the striving aspect of my twenty- and thirty-something life (it does seem like another life now), when I would try to calm that chaos with what most of us think we need in our younger decades: enough money, enough status, enough on our CV, enough clothes, enough scatter cushions, a kitchen island . . . all the stuff we think brings security and satisfaction. I have in fact just seen a video of people in their eighties and nineties saying exactly this – the 'stuff' they thought would make them happy didn't. Instead, what is important is how you lived and who you loved.

MDRC, if you like the idea of having some strings – some guidance, some calm, some freedom that comes from a total acceptance of who you are and what you are designed to be – then I hope these treasures can become that for you too.

If you stand on the foundation that your unique personhood and existence are utterly loved and approved, that who you are is to be honoured and dignified, then what you build will be beautiful and exciting and lasting.

You, and all you are, will never appear again in the history of humankind. Treasure you, please, thank you to you! You're a treasure. Okay, you get the point . . . Back to me . . . I was excited that the treasures I had peeled off the walls of the cave had become my strings. Each one a loving and gentle way to undo those patterns I needed to smash for a healthier existence. I had a clear new way. There was a manual!

The Armour Of Treasures

Don't isolate for fear of being misunderstood; armour with a safe ear to hear.

Let go of fixing and fighting and put on the armour of surrender, acceptance and trust.

Let go of invulnerability and pretence and put on the armour of allowing a full expression of emotions.

Avoid ignoring your thoughts; put on the armour of self-control, and learn not to believe the thoughts that cause you fear, filling yourself instead with the good that brings you peace.

Put on the armour of kindness and self-compassion so that you may meet your needs; say no, and state your preferences in order to love others better.

Guard yourself against the trap of achievement and look to find ways to honour your unique skills, talents and passions.

Respect yourself enough to rest and play, putting on the armour of joy.

Let go of pushing and rushing; listen to how you tick and put on the armour of gentleness to bring you firmly into the only moment you have: the present.

Put on the armour of patience, letting life unfold how it does, surrendering to and trusting the mystery of the highs and lows.

And most important of all, put on the armour of love.

Falling In Love

That list of the armour of treasures felt like it could be a perfect and poetic ending. But I'm back again! It's going to be hard to say goodbye to you, MDRC . . . Anyway, I couldn't end it there. I need to tell you whether the Hart heart finds love in the end.

Well, The Boy from Bristol did come back, and with something to share.

The being angry and grumpy didn't put him off. The body didn't put him off, despite witnessing some massive mid-life inflation my inner critic did not enjoy! The vulnerability didn't put him off. The talk of uncovering my wild self didn't put him off. None of my wildness put him off.

In fact, he came back to tell me he loved me.

Our time apart had shown us that we had indeed fallen hopelessly in love with each other.

Patti accepted and loved him. Peggy was looking down proud!

Yes, MDRC, The Boy became The Boyfriend. And never did I think I could ever meet anyone who could be so genuinely perfect for me in every way.

It was, as I have heard others say, like finding the missing piece of a jigsaw. One that I would regularly and infuriatingly search for, and then suddenly one day when I wasn't looking, I unexpectedly found it.

We started this story with the daring to listen to our longings. One of my deepest longings after isolation from illness was to find love. I remember hardly daring to admit that to myself. It meant I had to feel the pain of disconnection I was experiencing, the fear of a loving relationship not being fulfilled.

All I can say, MDRC, is if I hadn't dared to really admit what I wanted (within the boundaries of my values), it wouldn't have led to the grief that needed to pass to make way for the possibility. At the time, I had approximately 0.00001 per cent of hope that this longing could come to fruition. But . . . it was less than a year after that when I met The Boyfriend, and almost exactly a year after that, I was able to walk gently to the park hand in hand with him and do those things that make getting to know someone interesting and possible.

I'm not saying a romantic relationship is the answer. Your greatest longing might be for something else. It was love that I was ready for at that time in my life.

I remembered always wanting to get married at fifty-one. Perhaps I always instinctively knew that would be the right time.

Ummm . . . I wonder what might be in store . . . Steady Miranda, small steps . . .

I dared to say to him quite early on, 'When I am with you, I feel like I am home.' The feeling was reciprocated, though I would have been glad to have said it regardless. It's surely such a compliment to another that we should feel that safe and comfortable in their presence. It wasn't as if I needed him to 'come home' because I don't believe another person can ever complete us. I believe we must feel complete in ourselves. Falling in love can sometimes feel like a shortcut to a peace within ourselves as we are made to feel good by another, but if you can't feel that goodness without the compliments and the distraction of a heady honeymoon period, then it will be hard to sustain yourself or the relationship. Home is loving yourself as much as anyone else.

To that end I do think the treasures were ultimately a love letter to myself.

And because I had come home to myself, I was ready to love and be loved.

It's All Grace

I knew I was about to start again, from a different stance, and that the second half of my life would feel wholly different. At the same time, I didn't want to negate all that had come before.

I wrote down a list of moments from this unimportant yet significant life I had lived and was living; when it dawned on me that I had not been in control of pretty much any of it, I laughed. How grand we are to assume we are in control of most of our lives. How absurd that we try and control things we simply can't, get distressed when they don't go our way. I breathed a huge sigh of relief – I am not in control of much. What joy is this?!

Everything truly good in my life had been pure grace. The list was very, very long – I wrote everything down, from the fact that I was not in control of a dying woman sending me her book called *Call the Midwife* and saying it was being made for TV and she hoped I'd play Chummy, just as I am not in control of the creative ideas that come to me and what I am naturally good at. I was not in control of the fact that the woman who was going to take Peggy as a puppy broke her hip, so she was free for me to give her a home (the dog, not the woman.)

I will spare you the list of my life (although I recommend doing it) and give the one I have been dying to share:

I was not in control of the fact that I met my best friend and the love of my life who brings me more silliness, laughter, joy, support, care, safety than I thought possible in a person, because I lost my house due to mould illness and he was the building surveyor on the house remediation project.

Yes, MDRC, my love was Mr Mould Man! The one and the very same.

I am not saying that you need a mouldy house, or the equivalent, to find redemption in your life, but I do now believe that goodness can come from suffering.

May my Mr Mould Man / The Boy / The Boy from Bristol / The Boyfriend not just be a rom-com story, but both our ongoing hope, MDRC. Whenever I told any of my friends I had met someone, they all simply paused, confused, and said, 'HOW?!' It's not a high probability with housebound illness and a global pandemic for a knight in shining armour to appear on the doorstep. But he did. To de-mould me . . . (Stop it, we're better than that . . .)

The Same, But Different

When I took a taxi ride from one side of London to the other, seeing it for the first time in nearly seven years (this time asking confidently to sit in silence), I marvelled at both the mess and majesty of the city. I drove past many of the places I used to frequent, from glossy studios on the South Bank I performed in, to scruffy theatres I crewed in, to pubs and cafés I used to drink and gig in, to theatres I watched and acted in, to parks I walked in. It was all still there. The same, but different. I could say that for myself – I was the same, but different. Different because I felt solid, with a sense of wholeness.

I was no longer a pawn rocked by a city that was telling me what I should and shouldn't be doing, or wearing or saying, or how I should be functioning. I was not stuck in the whirlwind of a city's ways that scared or damaged me because I couldn't keep up or fit in. I felt calm and centred being away from that rat race and able to enjoy the city and all it had to offer knowing my little life was best served if I went about it simply, in the way I am wired and the way I tick.

When I think of the years gone by, I wish I hadn't struggled to learn what I needed to. If I'm honest, I wish never to feel physically and emotionally uncomfortable again. I wish my loved ones would never suffer. I wish I still didn't feel vulnerable and make mistakes. I wish I could just have a life of ease and joy. Those wishes were the same in the past. What is different is that I now know they are empty wishes. A life without those things doesn't exist, so the longing for them is forever painful. (Yes, we can get our longings wrong, so the guiding treasures remain ever important for me.)

We do not live in a trouble-free world. And more to the point, though it's often hard for our sensitive souls to hear, if it weren't for our darkness, our troubles, our suffering, we wouldn't necessarily become the strongest, wisest, calmest, most skilled version of ourselves. It can be what makes us, informs us, teaches us. It taught me not to waste precious life stuck in old patterns but to keep operating in line with my core identity.

Surely, the world's got it the wrong way round? We need to start at the end – believe in your inherent worth and beauty and you'll get up every morning with a smile on your face, excited about what you can bring to, learn from and develop for the world, for yourself and others, because you can't work your way into believing you are loved. God knows, most of us have tried.

What an assault not to consider ourselves a treasure this world needs. To hide ourselves. To fight to win love and therefore mask who we really are. May the treasures free you as they did me. You wild super elephant you!

In the taxi that day, I felt home in and with myself. I was in the city but separate from it. I had been undoing its patterns that had taken me away from my wild self and caused me pain. I said goodbye to the idea, once and for all and oh so very easily, that I could get comfort and security from the trappings of success, money, status, heightened experiences and that peculiar beast that is fame (let's remember fame is not our friend, children, unless a random by-product of your lovely honest selves).

Life was easier now.

I could enjoy the world because the world is not my home.

Home is inside, and home feels simple.

My Wild Secret

I am worthy, unique and wholly loved. Whatever you, I or anyone says.

I will try not to say sorry unless there's a need to apologize, and then my sorry is truly for you.

I am powerful, I am vulnerable.

I am strong, I am sensitive.

I am peaceful, I am passionate.

I am creative, I am efficient.

I am playful, I am pensive.

I am excitable and I have some wisdom.

I am adventurous and I like comfort.

I am productive and I am restful.

I have a strength I am shy about.

I am sensual.

I am athletic and wobbly.

I am awkward and elegant.

I try not to control, judge or fix, but I control, judge and fix.

I am self-aware!

I forgive when I am ready.

I am generous and I treat myself.

I do my best to love others as I would love to be loved.

I fail at that countlessly.

I am still loved.

I am changing and I am steadfast.

I am honest and I slip up.

I am whole.

I am free.

I am home.

I am me.

Picking Yourself Back Up

No, that wasn't the end either – I'm back AGAIN! I need to share with you something I found very profound, which will take us to our true goodbye.

An American friend of mine went to boarding school aged just eight. She has been haunted many times throughout her life by the image and feeling of being left in a large hallway of an imposing building, looking around to realize she could no longer see her parents, rushing upstairs to look for them, only to look out of a window and see their car turn out of the driveway and disappear. Emotionally that is very hard, or impossible, to understand aged eight – your safety and love suddenly torn away. You don't know that your mother is in floods of tears wondering what she has done, pulling over to decide whether to go back and get her daughter (as my friend later discovered, it being her grandparents who paid for her education and made the decision).

Decades after the event, this wound began to surface more regularly. She started to get many anxiety symptoms, and this anxiety manifested itself in a debilitating fear of letting her three daughters down or making wrong decisions for their lives. I told her that however 'wacky' it sounded, the science tells us that our brains lodge these memories and run strategies based off them. That part of the brain doesn't have a date stamp, so it doesn't realize the emotional reactions are in the past and not necessary now. The way to resolve that trauma is to feel the feelings of the hurt eight-year-old and go back and tell her that you are safe now. My friend looked at me perplexed. She was listening but didn't want to really hear it. Understandably. It sounds weird. It sounds hard. And it can be the latter.

A few months later we were talking about it again. One of her children had had a minor bullying incident at school, and she was having a panic attack that the incident might have lifelong repercussions. I gently showed her she was not acting like her adult self, and this was the eight-year-old wound playing out. She had a revelation as we talked it through. She realized that standing in that hall when she had seemingly been deserted way back in her past, she had made a clear decision. She was going to make sure that she and all her friends were going to be okay by controlling events as much as she could to make everyone feel happy and cosy. She wasn't going to let anything make her feel unsafe or alone. She started crying. 'There you go,' I told her. 'That's the root.'

At eight years old, she'd had to form a strategy to ease the agony of her source of safety and love being ripped from her. That's what we do when we've experienced trauma. We find the way to survive, and that pattern gets stuck throughout our lifetime. When we get older we slowly see that it's not helpful, and we discover what thoughts are running that are causing anxiety and unhelpful behaviours. The minute my friend saw this strategy, everything she was feeling many years on made sense. The love she had for her children was so strong, but the agony of them experiencing anything like she had meant she was controlling as much as she could about their lives. That was her cage. She began to regularly talk to that eight-year-old part of herself, telling her that she didn't need to be scared any more. Soon the control and fear lessened, and she could parent and love from a place of calm rather than terror of something going wrong. She was less tired, less anxious; she was freer and, simply, happier.

If we are lucky, and if we need to, we find where we have to go back to and pick ourselves up. Tell that part of

411

ourselves that we can change the way we operate now and move forward differently. Wildly.

Felled

Well, we really are coming to the end of our time together now, MDRC. A final little story to share.

I say that I have a, what I call, animal goof gene. You may have it too. It expresses itself when you see a cute animal and can't help but well up or feel such love for it you want to hold it so tightly it might burst. When you see an injured animal looking vulnerable on a wildlife programme and you know the likely outcome, you must leave the room until the predator has vanished, or the deed has been done. You simply can't cope with any form of animal cruelty or animal gorgeousness – both leave you a wreck of tears whether for pain or joy. That's the animal goof gene. I knew I had it when a limping seagull on a beach in Australia made me cry! A personality quirk I certainly am not in control of owning.

With that in mind, I therefore knew that watching horse racing was an absolute no-no for me. I know nothing of the sport; therefore I do nothing but project pain on to the horses as their gallops strain and their eyes become seemingly wide-eyed in terror as the jockey whips them to the finish line.

Yet, on an otherwise lovely April afternoon, I found myself in front of the television watching the Grand National. I was feeling a little on edge already because I was back in

Bristol – the city in which I made that decision to stay at university – for the first time in almost thirty years. I had just gone for a walk around the city centre, which included passing the Bristol Hippodrome. The theatre that I'd worked at, taking tickets and selling ice cream, before having to quit due to the first spate of hefty viral infections that rendered my energy too depleted to continue. This was of great disappointment at the time because the job at the Hippodrome was my remaining connection to my dream to be in theatre. It didn't matter that I was working front of house and not on or behind the stage. If I could be part of the magic of theatre by selling someone an ice cream at the interval, then I was happy (and yes, I did have a little tray with a strap around my shoulders, even a bow tie . . .).

I smiled at the young front of house staff outside the theatre the day I walked past, thinking of all the adventures ahead in their lives, whether they were longing to be actors, directors, stage managers or stay front of house, or whether it was just a job for now to fund the next step. I suddenly felt a well-known wave of grief hurtling towards me. A self-compassionate grief that at that time in my young life, it just hadn't ever worked out how I'd hoped and expected. Like life for so many, and far, far worse (I remain ever more awake to the perspective of my experience compared with so much deep tragedy we are surrounded by). It was grief from the memory of the first of many times I experienced being felled by illness that meant losing joy and aspects of my life that kept me afloat, content, connected to who I was.

I could see my twenty-year-old self in her bow tie and far too short skirt (it was the standard skirt length, I'm just tall – I wasn't hitching it up!), with her skinny athletic legs, slightly goofy posture, mouth wide open to breathe or to stare. I could see her sitting on her own at the back of the theatre watching the show (*Me and My Girl*) for the sixty-eighth time. I could feel the lightness in her body, the fizzing excitement of all the dreams. All in contrast to the heaviness of the grief forming in my now older and tired body.

I started to walk quickly back to where I was staying, where my loving boyfriend was watching the Grand National, and picked up the pace before the grief overwhelmed me on a busy city street. But I was bizarrely halted, on being recognized. Not bizarre that I was recognized but bizarre because it caused a full-circle life moment for me. A group of women about my age were getting out of a coach to see the show at the Hippodrome later that day. I heard a muttering of my name and a fizz of whispers going through their group.

In that moment I pictured my twenty-year-old self watching her fifty-year-old self. A little worried about her. Why was her head down, not upwards and smiling? And much more to the point, why were a group of women pointing at her?

Luckily the whole group didn't bombard me, and they didn't ask for selfies; instead, one person in the group came up to me (very close) and blew me a kiss (close enough for breath on face – thanks for that!) and said, 'We all love you so much, thank you.' And they screamed and bounced a bit, which my twenty-year-old self found VERY ODD.

As that kindly woman's breathy kiss faded away from my face, I gave them a quick smile and wave, and then bit my lip hard as the tears were close to uncontrollably falling. I also looked back at the Bristol Hippodrome and in my mind's eye waved goodbye to my jolly, bow-tied self. A bittersweet farewell, when despite knowing she would be excited by much of her next thirty years ahead, I also knew what she was going to have to go through.

By the time I got to The Boyfriend, the Grand National was about to begin, and the tears had dissipated. I didn't leave the room because I needed his company. He was my safe space. I briefly forgot the degree of the animal goof gene. That didn't last long because at the second or third fence, minutes into the race, I witnessed before my very eyes, seemingly in slow motion, a majestic creature fall at the fence after a dodgy jump and land on its neck, never to get up again.

The floodgates opened. I was heaving with grief, The Boyfriend a little startled, but happy to literally and metaphorically hold me in all the emotion that followed. The sadness of seeing that innocent, strong, stunning, wild, excited, hopeful creature in the prime of its life felled before my eyes was too much to bear. Which, in turn, released the pain of seeing my bow-tied young woman's wildness taken from her by illness and myriad other ensuing reasons.

Despite the sadness, the tears slowly metamorphosed from deep grief into the relief that I was fully free again for the first time in those thirty years. My wildness was returning, whether fully physically healed yet or not.

But I needed to do one more thing. I knew where I had to go back to and pick myself up from.

The Final Hello

It was time for me to heed the advice I'd given my friend who had suffered the boarding school trauma. I was to go back, in my mind, to greet my nineteen-year-old self at baggage reclaim before she got to university and became sick. So I went back to that dreary, grey, strip-lit part of the airport and sat down and held her hand. I told her that I understood what she was feeling. And that she was right. She was indeed becoming caged, losing herself. I thanked her because if she hadn't felt those things then, I wouldn't be listening acutely now. I told her that it was finished. I had set myself free of the worldly rules that had fully caged her. I hugged her and told her I had remembered the parts of her that I had lost, that had been pushed down to conform. And I was reclaiming them.

I told her she wasn't making up any of the symptoms she had been experiencing, and her instinct was right about the anxiety diagnoses never matching – it was in fact a tick-borne illness. I told her it wasn't her fault she was going to have to walk through the arrivals gate, as there was no other option. But it was okay because now I don't need to be in the Australian outback to be at home in myself.

I picked up that nineteen-year-old's rucksack, threw thirty years of emotional baggage to circulate in that stuffy airport baggage reclaim and end up in lost property, never to be reclaimed, took her by the hand and walked towards the sliding doors knowing that I had learnt all I needed to be free. That she was once again her true, wild, uncaged self. We were home.

I looked her in the eye and smiled. 'Better late than never,' I said. She smiled back. 'Where are we going?' she asked. 'To a bluebell wood,' I replied. We skipped into the arrivals hall with a new rucksack. One full of the treasures from our darkness.

P.S. I Haven't Been Entirely Honest . . .

An extraordinary day on an ordinary January day.

The Boyfriend suggested we go to Kew Gardens for a walk. It was a delightful potter and became rather magical when the sun started to break through grey clouds as we approached a wide, winding bridge across a lake. I felt The Boyfriend squeeze my hand, which usually meant he was feeling emotional about the beauty of something. That was true, but it turned out his heart was starting to race for another reason. We stood still on the bridge overlooking the lake when the silence was pierced as he rather seriously said, 'Miranda.' I turned around, and as I did, he got down on one knee. 'Miranda . . .'

I don't remember anything else because I simply burst out crying, apparently saying yes before he had finished the sentence (awkward if he'd been tying a shoelace . . .). For the slower among you . . . he was asking me to marry him. Are you with us?! Hello?!!

I didn't think a traditional proposal would affect me so. But there was someone knowing all my ridiculousness and brokenness and still willing to bend down, look up and commit to loving me and standing by me for the rest of his life.

417

I was immediately back in airport arrivals, telling the young me that it may have taken me three decades to pick her up, and I will always hold sadness that it took that long, but we really could now move the story onward. A marriage to a kind, loving and really fun (almost as silly as me!) man; but as importantly, a marriage of all the treasures I had learnt to my young self's joy, dreams and energy to live authentically. That's wild.

So, I wasn't *entirely* honest . . .

He's not my boyfriend.

He's my husband.

We got married when I was fifty-one.

Recommended Reading

MDRC, if you are feeling like your life needs some change but feel lost as to where to begin (as I was), here are some of the key books that I read. I hope they might help develop the treasures for you.

The list could be very long indeed, but below are a wide variety that I do believe can help guide us towards the peaceful living we are designed for.

I have felt held, nurtured, understood, relieved, encouraged and inspired by them all. And they predominantly have simple, practical and fun application to the reasoning behind them.

I am sure you will get a sense of what books feel right for you at specific times, and simply delving in with some of these will begin that process and lead you to others. Most of these people also have fantastic online and free resources to listen to and watch.

Martha Beck, *Finding Your Own North Star: How to Claim the Life You Were Meant to Live*, London: Piatkus, 2003.
Martha is a sociologist and bestselling author, and has been through it all herself. These help us to understand how our particular fears hold us back and help to uncover who we

really are and how we want to live our lives with unique purpose.

Byron Katie, *Loving What Is: Four Questions That Can Change Your Life*, London: Rider, 2002.

Byron Katie went from alcoholism, agoraphobia and rage to pure enlightenment in an instant as she suddenly saw thoughts for what they are. She realized that what she was believing was causing her suffering, nothing more. Her work is particularly good for relationships, but works on all. Visit her website, www.thework.com, *for all* things Byron Katie.

Anne Lamott, *Help, Thanks, Wow*, London: Hodder & Stoughton, 2013.

Anne is a beautiful writer with huge life experience, and this simple book will feel like a hug as you are gently being told, 'It's all going to be okay'.

Steven Hayes and Spencer Smith, *Get Out of Your Mind and Into Your Life*, Oakland: New Harbinger Publications, 2005.

Steven is a psychologist, but this is easy to read and practical, as he formed a therapeutic approach from his own experiences. If you are beginning to acknowledge unhealthy thought patterns, anxiety or phobias, it's a great step to work on those and is wholly curative if applied.

Mark Williams and Danny Penman, *Mindfulness: A Practical Guide to Finding Peace in a Frantic World*, London: Piatkus, 2011.

The definitive mindfulness book. A route to acceptance and surrender. It comes with short guided meditations too.

Vidyamala Burch and Danny Penman, *Mindfulness for Health: A Practical Guide to Relieving Pain, Reducing Stress and Restoring Wellbeing*, **London: Piatkus, 2013.**

This one is specifically focused on acceptance for chronic health issues. Vidyamala Burch has a website that has affordable online courses and meditations for people living with chronic illness, www.breathworks-mindfulness.org.uk.

Simon Sinek, *Find your Why: A Practical Guide for Discovering Purpose for You and Your Team*, **London: Penguin, 2017.**

A practical guide for discovering purpose and finding fulfillment at work. He also has a course on his website, www.simonsinek.com.

Maria Forleo, *Everything is Figureoutable*, **London: Penguin Business, 2019.**

A simple read on discovering purpose, more specifically about how to turn your ideas and passions into a reality, overcoming imposter syndrome, procrastination, etc.

Pia Mellody, Andrea Wells Miller and J. Keith Miller, *Facing Codependence: What It Is, Where It Comes from, How It Sabotages Our Lives*, **San Francisco: Harper Collins, 2003.**

If you want to understand people-pleasing tendencies, how to meet your needs, and why it's important for your relationships and general wellbeing, this will uncover that for you. There is also an accompanying workbook, *Breaking Free: A Recovery Workbook for Facing Codependence*.

Viktor E. Frankl, *Man's Search for Meaning*, London: Rider, 2004.

If you want a story as well as an inspiring way to look at your life (and some anxiety cures) from a psychologist who survived the holocaust, then look no further. You could also read *The Choice* by **Edith Eger**. Incredible.

Anything by Brené Brown

Braving the Wilderness or *Rising Strong* might be good ones to start with. If you haven't listened to her Ted Talks on vulnerability and shame, please google forthwith. I think of all her books *The Gifts of Imperfection* might relate most to the treasures.

Parker J. Palmer, *Let Your Life Speak*, San Francisco: John Wiley & Sons, 2000.

An essay more than a book, so a nice easy read. Palmer is a Quaker who inspires what our unique vocation is and talks honestly and beautifully about his periods of depression.

Dr Caroline Leaf, *The Perfect You Workbook: A Blueprint for Identity*, Michigan: Baker Books, 2018.

If you need science, Caroline Leaf will have many, many books for you. She is a neuroscientist and it's her mission to spread the truth that we can change how our brain is wired and move away from negativity bias. This one is a little heavy – it matches science with the Bible (she has others just from a secular perspective that are a little simper) – but I found it mindblowing to see how we are wired uniquely and not meant to operate from any kind of fear, scientifically and spiritually. If you work through her questionnaire, you learn huge amounts about yourself and how you tick.

Elaine Aron, *The Highly Sensitive Person: How to Thrive When the World Overwhelms You*, London: Thorsons, 2017.
This, alongside **Susan Cain's** Ted Talk 'The Power of Introverts' and her book *Quiet*, has given me an understanding of how to nurture a more sensitive soul, and more to the point, that it is fine to be one!

Richard Rohr, *Immortal Diamond: The Search for Our True Self*, London: SPCK Publishing, 2013.
Richard is an academic and a Catholic Mystic so his books are meaty. Although I don't have an academic brain, I was captivated by this book. It's about what our souls, or True Selves, are, and how we sleepwalk through life operating from our False Selves, or egos. When the True Self drives the ship, then you are in peace and joy.

Jeffrey E. Young and Janet S. Klosko, *Reinventing Your Life*, London: Scribe, 2019.
Another one for those who want a therapy approach. Whereas Steven Hayes's book has a more practical application of anxiety and phobias, this book focuses on emotional root causes of suffering. There are quizzes (I love a quiz!) to help you uncover some patterns you may not know you have.

Susan David, *Emotional Agility: Get Unstuck, Embrace Change, and Thrive in Work and Life*, London: Penguin Life, 2016.

So good and simple on emotions and some great self-compassion insight.

Stuart Brown, M.D., with Christopher Vaughan, *Play: How it Shapes the Brain, Opens the Imagination, and Invigorates the Soul*, New York: Avery, 2010.

Does what it says on the tin – teaches you all about play, and how it is a vital necessity to put back into and keep in our lives.

Charles Duhigg, *The Power of Habit: Why We Do What We Do, and How to Change*, London: Penguin, 2013.

Changing your life by looking at your daily habits and how they are formed. *Atomic Habits* **by James Clear** is also great, all about tiny changes making the long-term, massive difference. If you like loud, motivating personal speaker-type stuff then **Tony Robbins** might be for you.

John E. Sarno M.D., *The Divided Mind: The Epidemic of Mindbody Disorders*, London: Duckworth, 2024.

If you suffer from confusion or even cynicism, and need some scientific proof of the mind-body connection, then delve into this, or *The Body Keeps the Score* **by Bessel van der Kolk.** Our bodies truly are a mirror of our mind. They are our greatest teacher, yet we ignore them, override and berate them, which is when problems can arise. **Alex Howard's** *It's Not Your Fault* would be a great one, too – especially if you have ME/CFS.

Dr Will Cole, *The Inflammation Spectrum*: *Find Your Food Triggers and Reset Your System*, London: Hodder & Stoughton, 2023.

This contains some practical lifestyle tips to help the body reduce inflammation including food suggestions. It can lead to changes in things that you may have accepted to be part of your life, from tiredness and brain fog to IBS, rashes and pain.

Acknowledgements

I often read acknowledgements in a book, but I'm not entirely sure why! Perhaps I read them in books I have truly loved, to savour their every and final word. Sometimes a book can become such a friend that I don't want it to end, and the acknowledgements are the last tiny remnants of my relationship with the author. Sometimes I hope they might give me a little peek into the author's private life, or that I could miraculously know someone they have thanked, so there's a chance I could become their best friend!

That propels me to acknowledge the bold, brilliant, beautiful women who I have been inspired by and learnt so much from. The list could be very long indeed, but the ones who particularly helped me in recent years, and to whom I am deeply grateful for their work are: Brené Brown, Caroline Leaf, Sue Monk Kidd, Martha Beck, Edith Eger and Byron Katie. They are very much part of the treasures. And I very much want to be their best friend . . .

Someone who is already a best friend and introduced me to other greats like Elizabeth Gilbert, Tara Brach, Ellen Langer, Maya Angelou and Mary Oliver is genius (truly) storyteller Julia Voce. Thank you, Jools, for your friendship in the hard times, for loving Peggy and Patti (!) and for reading an early draft of the book, bravely shouting at times 'don't understand' or 'bored now'. This book needed that expert candour and wisdom! That's honest friendship.

I want to thank my sister and the group of friends who surprised me on my fiftieth birthday with a list of words they felt encapsulated me. A risk – I think one person did put 'windy' – but it was one of the most wonderful gifts I have ever been given; sowing the seed of how we are identified beyond worldly measures, and an encouragement that my story and what I had learnt was worth telling. Forever grateful.

Thank you to the wise and kind people who gave their time to read the book before publication – Jo Rice, Jess Thompson, Pete Grieg, Alice Goodwin-Hudson, Sydney Jenkins, Rose Heiney, Simon Sinek and Christine Dunkley. Your thoughts were hugely helpful and encouraging. And thank you to Mo Vernon who wrote up all my endless research notes all those years ago. Mo, you helped me kick-start the long process. And Emma Abrahams (watch this space for her name as an actor) – you helped me to be able to finish it, with your literal and metaphorical neighbourly care and love, as well as your efficient admin assistance. (And let's never forget it was you who came up with the bestselling 'I bloody love crisps' bowl and pen at The Miranda Shop – genius!)

There have been many wonderful doctors and practitioners who didn't 'tatt' me about. I won't say your full names here, for you may get inundated, but thank you Debbie, Laura, Michael, Louise, Peg, Amelia, Jennifer, Jess, Sarah, Ed, Alan and John.

Finally, there are two men without whom this book wouldn't exist. The Boy, or rather The Husband, who listened with patience and kindness not only to sections of the book, but to the moanings of the process and worries of not getting it done. And made me countless meals and snacks along the way to keep me going. Husband – you are, truly, the greatest gift of my life (not just for the meals and snacks). You gave me my joy back.

And then there's my agent, Gordon Wise at Curtis Brown. He has been one of the most loyal, patient and kind people in my professional life, sticking by me through all the very difficult ups and downs of illness, and not letting go before I had a diagnosis and the possibility of recovery to work again. Thank you, Gordon.

And thank you for daring to send publishing goddess Louise Moore my not always great poems to see what she thought. Thank you, Louise, for not knowing anything about poetry and whether they were good or bad (your words) and daring to have a meeting about whether I could share my story! And thank you, Louise, for introducing me to editor extraordinaire Jill Taylor, who helped my ramblings and research make sense (no mean feat – Jill, you have an amazing brain I am grateful to have plundered!) And thank you, for laughing with me along the way and encouraging me by sharing that the treasures helped you (oh, and advising me on shoes and shirts!) Thank you so much, Louise and Jill, and your team at Penguin, for helping to facilitate getting back to work for the first time in a while could work alongside my ongoing recovery. I am truly grateful.

I have understood through this process, more than in any other, the vital need for connection and support to help each other be the best of ourselves. I will never 'go it alone' again.

Text Permissions

Part One: Trapped

p.12 – Ware, B. (2012), *The Top Five Regrets of the Dying*, Hay House.

p.24 – Eger, E. (2017), *The Choice: A True Story of Hope*, Rider.

Treasure One: Share

p.45 – Buechner, F. (1991), *Telling Secrets: A Memoir*, HarperSanFrancisco.

p.47 – Brown, B. (2020), *The Gifts of Imperfection*, Vermillion.

p.61 – Boyle, G. (2017), *Barking to the Choir: The Power of Radical Kinship*, Simon & Schuster.

Treasure Two: Surrender

p.71 – Williams, M. & Penman, D. (2011), *Mindfulness: A Practical Guide to Finding Peace in a Frantic World*, Piatkus.

pp.83 – 4 – Gordon, A. (2020), *The Way Out: The Revolutionary, Scientifically Proven Approach to Heal Chronic Pain*, Vermillion.

p.93 – Monk, S. (2006), *When the Heart Waits: Spiritual Direction for Life's Sacred Questions*, Bravo Ltd.

Treasure Four: Thoughts

pp.151 – 2 – Milne, A. A. (2016), *The House at Pooh Corner*, Copyright © Pooh Properties Trust 1928. Reproduced with permissions from Curtis Brown Group Ltd on behalf of The Pooh Properties Trust.

p.154 – Rinpoche, Y. M. (2019), In Love with the World: *What a Buddhist Monk Can Teach You About Living from Nearly Dying*, Bluebird.

p.169 – Turner, T. (2020), *Happiness Becomes You: A Guide to Changing Your Life for Good*, Harper Collins.

p.170 – Katie, B. (2002), *Loving What Is: Four Questions That Can Change Your Life*, Harmony.

Treasure Five: Loving Ourselves

pp.185 – 6 – Rohr, R. (2018), 'Walking Toward Heaven,' *Richard Rohr's Daily Meditations*, June 21, 2018. Copyright © 2018 by CAC. Used by permission of CAC. All rights reserved worldwide.

p.194 – Neff, K. (2011), *Self-Compassion: Stop Beating Yourself Up and Leave Insecurity Behind*, William Morrow & Co.

p.203 – Palmer, P. J. (1999), *Let Your Life Speak: Listening for the Voice of Vocation*, Jossey Bass.

p.208 – Mellody, P. (2002), *Facing Codependence: What It Is, Where It Comes from, How It Sabotages Our Lives*, HarperOne.

pp.219 – 21 – Aron, E. (1997), *The Highly Sensitive Person: How to Thrive When the World Overwhelms You*, Harmony.

Treasure Six: Why We Do, What We Do

p.226 – 'Heigh-Ho' written by Frank Churchill (music) and Larry Morey (lyrics).

p.237 – Palmer, P. J. (1999), *Let Your Life Speak: Listening for the Voice of Vocation*, Jossey Bass.

p.249 – Hayes, S. (2005), *Get Out of Your Mind and Into Your Life: The New Acceptance & Commitment Therapy*, New Harbinger Publications.

p.249 – David, S. (2016), *Emotional Agility: Get Unstuck, Embrace Change, and Thrive in Work and Life*, Avery Publishing Group.

p.254 – Lamott, A. (1995), *Bird by Bird: Some Instructions on Writing and Life*, Vintage/ Penguin Random House.

Treasure Seven: Play

p.265 – Brown, S. (2009), *Play: How It Shapes the Brain, Opens the Imagination, and Invigorates the Soul*, Avery Publishing Group.

p.283 – Tree, I. (2018),*Wilding: The Return of Nature to a British Farm*, Picador Books/ Pan Macmillan.

p.285 – Scott Kortge, C. (2010), *Healing Walks For Hard Times: Quiet Your Mind, Strengthen Your Body, and Get Your Life Back*, Shambala.

Treasure Eight: Pacing and Presence

p.308 – Burch, V. and Penman, D. (2013), *Mindfulness for Health: A Practical Guide to Relieving Pain, Reducing Stress and Restoring Wellbeing*, Hachette.

p.310 – Lieberman, C. (2018), 'How Self-Care Became So Much Work', *Harvard Business Review*.

p.319 – Keller, T. (2021), 'Growing My Faith in the Face of Death', *The Atlantic*.

p.322 – Clear, J. (2018), *Atomic Habits: Tiny Changes, Remarkable Results*, Random House Business.

Treasure Nine: Don't Fear the Setback

p.361 – Handler, D. (2001), *The Ersatz Elevator (A Series of Unfortunate Events)*, HarperCollins Childrens.

Treasure Ten: It's All About Love in the End

p.382 – Hayes, S. (2019), *A Liberated Mind: The Essential Guide to ACT*, Vermillion.

p.383 – Baldwin, J. (1990), *The Fire Next Time*, Penguin Classics.

p.385 – Brown, B. (2015), *Daring Greatly: How the Courage to Be Vulnerable Transforms the Way We Live, Love, Parent, and Lead*, Penguin Life.

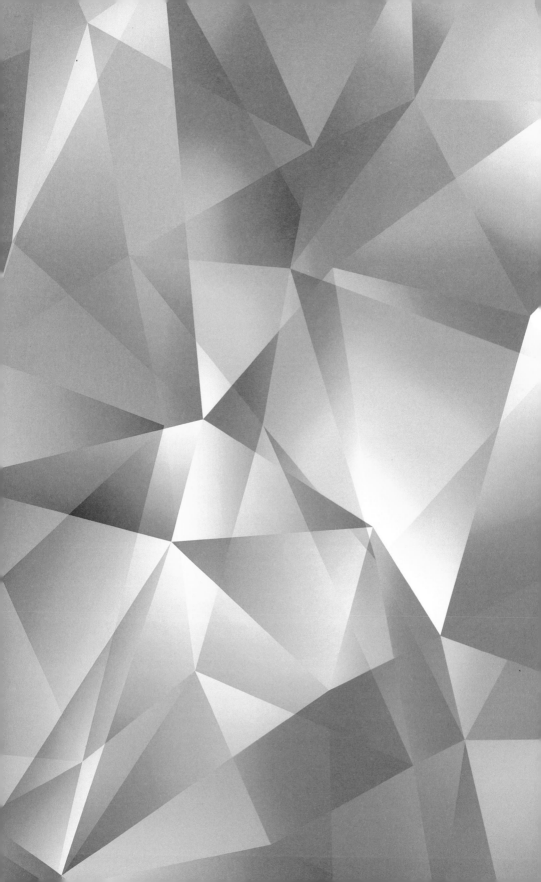